ULTIMATE STRENGTH TRAINING GUIDE FOR SENIORS OVER 60

DISCOVER HOW ADULTS OVER 60 CAN REGAIN STRENGTH AND BALANCE TO LIVE A HAPPIER, HEALTHIER LIFE

MELANIE DAHN, MSN, APRN-NPC

© **Copyright 2023 - All rights reserved.**

The content contained within this book may not be reproduced, duplicated or transmitted without direct written permission from the author or the publisher.

Under no circumstances will any blame or legal responsibility be held against the publisher, or author, for any damages, reparation, or monetary loss due to the information contained within this book, either directly or indirectly.

Legal Notice:

This book is copyright protected. It is only for personal use. You cannot amend, distribute, sell, use, quote or paraphrase any part, or the content within this book, without the consent of the author or publisher.

Disclaimer Notice:

Please note the information contained within this document is for educational and entertainment purposes only. All effort has been executed to present accurate, up to date, reliable, complete information. No warranties of any kind are declared or implied. Readers acknowledge that the author is not engaged in the rendering of legal, financial, medical or professional advice. The content within this book has been derived from various sources. Please consult a licensed professional before attempting any techniques outlined in this book.

By reading this document, the reader agrees that under no circumstances is the author responsible for any losses, direct or indirect, that are incurred as a result of the use of the information contained within this document, including, but not limited to, errors, omissions, or inaccuracies.

CONTENTS

Introduction	5
1. IS THIS THE BODY I KNEW?	9
What's Happening to My Body?	10
Are These Health Issues Familiar?	16
2. WHY STRENGTH TRAIN?	25
What's Strength Training?	29
Why Do You Need Strength Training—12 Reasons	36
Don't Believe These!	41
Achieve a Strong Body With These Tips	43
Where's the Motivation?—Overcome the Barriers	46
3. KICKSTART YOUR JOURNEY	53
Start With the Equipment	54
What Should I Wear?	60
Your Rulebook to Safety	63
Why Stretch Before and After Your Workout?	68
Warming Up and Cooling Down	70
Reps and Rest in Strength Training	77
4. CHEST EXERCISES	79
The Chest Anatomy	80
Let's Begin!	81
5. STRENGTHEN YOUR SHOULDERS AND ARMS	87
The Shoulder and Arm Anatomy	87
Arm Exercises	89
Shoulder Exercises	95
6. LEG, ANKLES, AND FEET EXERCISES	101
The Leg Anatomy	101
Exercises You Should Try	103

7. LET'S STRENGTHEN THE BACK 115
   The Back Anatomy 115
   Lower Back Exercises 117
   Upper Back Exercises 125

8. BUILD YOUR STRENGTH, FROM THE CORE . . . 131
   The Core Anatomy 132
   Exercises You Should Try 133

9. THE ABDOMINALS 145
   The Abdominal Anatomy 145
   Exercises You Should Try 146

   Conclusion 157
   References 161

INTRODUCTION

> *There's no such thing as aging but maturing and knowledge. It's beautiful, I call that beauty.*
>
> — CELINE DION

As people age, they must undergo several changes in their bodies. One of the most striking changes is the involuntary loss of muscle function, strength, and mass. This process is termed sarcopenia (Evans, 1995). Did you know that once you have reached the age of 30, the decrease rate of muscle mass can be as much as 3–8% every ten years? (Holloszy, 2000). Yes, and after the age of 60, this rate increases even further. We often see older adults falling prey to a disability, and this loss of muscle mass is the leading cause of that.

If you have purchased this book, I understand that you probably fear losing your independence and relying on others to perform simple tasks like showering or getting to the toilet. You are witnessing your body becoming stiff and painful, making you immobile. Hence, you are looking for ways to improve mobility and strengthen your body muscles since you don't like the feeling of weakness that comes with aging. If all this seems relatable, then you have come to the perfect place because, in this book, we will talk about the benefits of physical activity and targeted strength training for seniors that can keep sarcopenia at bay.

Are you no longer feeling steady? Are your feet becoming less steady, making you worried about falls and injuries in the house? Do you always live in fear of falling and breaking your bones? Don't worry because a study conducted on older adults showed that low-intensity strength training and walking could have a major impact on disability problems and, in fact, reduce the risk of mobility being limited (Fielding et al., 2017).

Because of all the body changes that come with aging, people often develop low self-esteem. They avoid social places or meeting up with their friends because they feel that their appearance and deteriorating health makes them appear unattractive. This is especially the case for menopausal women. They understand the importance of regular strength training exercises, but they feel demotivated to start the programs or don't believe strength training is also fit for seniors. Their health conditions are also responsible for preventing or demotivating them from strength training. They also don't know the right exercises and how much exercise they need. But if you want to improve your quality of life, this book has just what you have been looking for. It will not only help you to reduce your physical vulnerability but also build resilience and keep chronic illnesses as far away as possible or at least manage them effectively.

Some of the things that you will learn from reading this book are how to feel stronger for longer, how to decrease fall-related injuries, tips to increase your balance and strength, and essential stretches for a full-body warm-up and cool-down. You will also learn some easy strength training exercises for major muscle groups without the need to leave your homes.

Now, since you will be bearing with me throughout this book, I thought that it's best I introduce myself to you and explain why I decided to write this book. My name is Melanie Dahn, and I am a 59-year-old, board-certified family nurse practitioner (MSN, APRN-C) with over ten years of experience and a passion for health, wellness, and disease prevention. I enjoy teaching health and wellness to the elderly, as well as others. I have helped many seniors learn to gain mobility and strength. I hope that by sharing my knowledge, I will empower readers to feel in control of their bodies and manage the effects of aging on their muscle mass and strength.

If you are just getting started on this journey, I must admit that in the beginning, it might not be easy, but at the same time, it need not be complicated or scary, as you will see in this book. Remember that something is always better than nothing, so if you have missed a session or two in the initial days, don't beat yourself up for it. Instead, make a promise to show up the next day. Including strength training in your routine is a lifestyle change, and it's like a marathon, not a sprint—you will have to keep doing it for long-term results and not give up in between.

Since you have already decided to purchase this book, this was your first step towards a better lifestyle. Keep in mind that in strength training for seniors, the end results are marvelous, even though the time commitment is low. In this book, you will find safe and efficient exercises that will help you get started and function more effectively throughout the rest of your life. All you need to keep in mind is that you must get your physician's approval and then stick to the recommendations. So, without any further ado, let's dive right in!

1

IS THIS THE BODY I KNEW?

> *Determined, dedicated, disciplined; that's what it takes to be fit, and to do strength training at any age. You can't give up, you have to keep going, and never let age be an excuse.*
>
> — ERNESTINE SHEPHERD

As we age, our bodies undergo some inevitable changes. These changes can be seen in muscle loss, joint and bone deterioration, and alterations to our body shape. While it can sometimes be difficult to accept these changes, they are a normal part of the aging process that cannot be avoided and should not be feared. Instead, it is important for us to understand why these changes occur so we may learn how to enable healthy aging and maintain overall physical health throughout our lives. This chapter discusses body changes that happen as people age and the health issues seniors experience. It analyzes muscle loss, the effect of aging on bones and joints, and body shape.

WHAT'S HAPPENING TO MY BODY?

Your body is made up of water, bones, lean tissue, and fat tissue, but after a person has reached the age of 30, the percentage of lean tissue in the body starts to decline. Your kidney, liver, muscles, and some other organs lose their cells. This process is termed atrophy (Lexell et al., 1988). There will be a lot of things that will be different about your body, but this is just part of the aging process and is completely normal. Some of the changes might be noticeable instantly, while some go unnoticed for a long period of time. If you want to be more aware of your body, here's a breakdown of everything that happens during this time.

Bones and Joints

Both men and women will experience a decrease in bone density after the age of 30. The deterioration of the function, structure, and composition of bones as you age is the previous stage of osteoporosis, which can be prevented if you take the necessary steps. Your body has its own cycle of bone resorption and bone formation so that the old bone cells can be replaced with new ones to enhance strength and durability. But this balance is often unsettled when a person starts aging, and the rate of bone resorption becomes more than bone formation (Demontiero et al., 2012). This, in turn, leads to reduced strength, osteoporosis, and insufficiency fractures.

As you may know, cartilage is the cushion-like tissue present between bones that assists in smooth movements. But as you age, you face flexibility issues, and your joints become increasingly stiffer. The reason behind this is that the cartilage starts to become thin, and there is a decrease in the synovial fluid present within the synovial joints of the body. The ligaments also lose flexibility as they become shortened, making your joints feel even stiffer (Better Health Channel, n.d.).

Another age-related change that you should be aware of after the age of 25 is the decline in the levels of collagen. Collagen is responsible for the flexibility in your skeletal system, and thus, when its levels drop, your bones become brittle and stiff (Bailey, n.d.).

Muscles and Body Fat

As already stated in the introduction, the loss of muscle function that happens due to aging is termed sarcopenia. To some extent, muscle loss would not affect your body fatally, but if 40% of the lean muscle mass of the body is lost, then it can be fatal to your survival (Roubenoff & Castaneda, 2001). But did you know that even though sarcopenia may be a universal problem, it doesn't affect all races and gender equally? (Noto et al., 2022). In fact, it has also been found that if you have any respiratory disease, diabetes mellitus, dementia, or cardiovascular disease, then you will have a higher chance of developing sarcopenia (Pacifico et al., 2020). With age, the number of muscle fibers in the body also decreases, which, in turn, reduces your strength (Henwood et al., 2008). On the other hand, the reduced muscle mass in the body is replaced by connective tissue and fat, both of which are noncontractile structures.

Skin

It's probably no secret that with age, the skin undergoes a huge change that is also visible to the naked eye. What might first look like a little discoloration here and there and a few fine lines underneath your eye, eventually become significant changes. When you reach your 40s, that's when the real change to the firmness of the skin starts. You will find it becoming saggy, which is mainly because of a loss in elasticity and volume. You will also notice more prominent sun damage and wrinkles at this age. In your youth, your skin was probably more radiant and had a dewy appearance, but as you age, that is going to fade away, paving the way for a duller complexion. This is mainly because the levels of moisture in the skin start to decrease with age. Your skin also looks less plump because of the loss of fat from the subcutaneous layer.

Once you have reached the age of 50, one of the most evident things you will see about your skin is bone loss, which affects the region around the skin, leading to puckering of the skin. The bony features of the nose also become more visible mainly due to the loss of cartilage in the area.

In women, changes take place a little bit differently as they undergo menopause around the age of 50. There is a major shift in the hormones in their bodies, whereby the level of androgens start increasing, and on the other hand, the estrogen levels take a dip. This is also a reason behind losing the elasticity of the skin and dryness, which in turn can lead to acne in some women (Corpuz, 2023).

Brain and Nervous System

Did you know that your nervous system and your brain also undergo several changes as you age? And these changes are completely natural! Once you have reached a certain age, brain function starts to follow a downward path (Maiese, 2020). The chances of developing dementia, white matter lesions, and stroke increase as you age, along with fluctuations in hormone and neurotransmitter levels, which can also cause memory impairment.

Once you reach the age of 40, approximately 5% of brain weight reduces every decade, mostly because of neuronal loss (Svennerholm et al., 1997). It has also been found, especially in people who develop problems like Alzheimer's, that it leads to the formation of tiny, discolored areas in the brain. This is because of the deposition of neuromelanin or black pigments and lipofuscin or brown pigments (Knight & Nigam, 2017).

With age, pathogens are also able to attack the brain more easily because of the weakening blood-brain barrier. According to research, the weakening often starts first in the hippocampus region, which is why many people suffer from cognitive decline in old age (Montagne et al., 2015). Moreover, by the time a person reaches the age of 70, cerebral blood flow is reduced almost by 27% (Chen et al., 2011). If someone suffers from atherosclerosis, especially in the arteries that supply blood to the brain, then cerebral blood flow decreases at an even faster rate.

As you age, the nervous system also weakens, which can lead to a loss of sensation in several parts of the body. Moreover, the disks that are present in between the vertebrae are no longer as flexible as they used to be, and as a result, the vertebrae sometimes overgrow. More pressure starts developing on the spinal cord because the disks are now not able to provide sufficient cushioning. At the same time, the nerves that emerge from the spinal cord also must endure increased pressure, which injures fibers in them to the extent that they leave the spinal cord. This type of injury often leads to a decrease in balance and strength.

The peripheral nerves of the body also become weak and are not able to transmit reflexes the way they used to before, which is what makes older people clumsier (Maiese, 2020).

Endocrine System

Most of the hormones in our body decrease in levels as we age, but there are some that are supposed to remain at the same level throughout our lives, irrespective of our age. However, even then, there are irregularities in the endocrine system due to age because if the hormone levels themselves do not fluctuate, the hormone receptors gradually lose their sensitivity (Young, 2022).

For example, the beta cells present in your pancreas lose their secretory capacity, and thus, as people age, their glucose tolerance no longer remains the same. Similarly, thyroid function, as well as pituitary activity, are also affected. Some of the common hormones that reduce with age are melatonin, growth hormone, and testosterone in men and estrogen in women.

Body Shape

It's very normal for your body to change in shape as you age. Do you know why? Well, as you learned in the previous paragraphs, your bones, joints, muscles, and fats are changing. These form the structure of your body, so your appearance is bound to change. It's true that aging causes a loss in bones and muscles, but simultaneously, you gain fat, and most of this fat is accumulated in the abdominal region alone. People also become shorter with age. Once a person reaches the age of 40, they usually lose approximately one centimeter every decade. After the age of 70, this loss in height becomes even more prominent and rapid.

The body shape changes also vary between men and women. Men mostly gain weight until they have reached the age of 55, and after that, they witness a reduction in body weight. Some say that this might be related to the dropping levels of testosterone around the same time. For women, the numbers are slightly different. They continue gaining weight until about 65, after which is a downward curve for them too.

Now that you are familiar with how aging affects different parts of your body, we will move on to some common health problems you should be aware of, especially when you approach senior life.

ARE THESE HEALTH ISSUES FAMILIAR?

It's a no-brainer that your body is going to be affected by different types of health issues with age, but if you are wary of these common ailments, it will help you have the upper hand on them. In this section, we are going to talk about some of the common health concerns that everyone should know about as they age because a healthy diet, proper sleep, and regular exercise can help you manage all of them.

Heart Disease

Let's first have a look at how your heart health changes with age. Anyone aged 65 and above is more susceptible to suffering from heart failure, coronary artery disease, stroke, and heart attack (National Institute on Aging, n.d.). However, for women, this age is 72 (How Aging Affects Your Heart, n.d.). Women also undergo menopause around the age of 50, leading to a decrease in estrogen levels. Now you might be wondering why I am mentioning this and what this has to do with heart health. I'll break it down for you. Estrogen is responsible for maintaining the flexibility of the arteries, so naturally, when its levels drop, the risk of heart attack rises (Khalil, 2013).

Another significant change your body goes through as you age is a decrease in metabolism. In fact, it can decrease by as much as 30% by the time a person reaches the age of 50 (Raman, 2017). However, these effects can be reduced with the help of strength training, as you will learn throughout this book. But a slower metabolism means that it will be even more challenging for you to maintain your weight in the healthy range. This further increases the risk of obesity, high blood pressure, and high cholesterol—all of which are linked with a rise in the risk of heart disease.

With age, the arteries of your cardiovascular system lose their flexibility and become stiff (Kohn et al., 2015). The muscles of your heart also become hardened, and together, it makes it difficult for the heart to pump blood to different parts of your body.

Moreover, aging disrupts your sleep cycle, and because of this, you tend to get less sleep. Poor sleep quality can harden the cholesterol plaque in arteries (Paddock, 2019). This increases the chances of heart attacks. People over the age of 50 also experience broken heart syndrome, which is where they experience shortness of breath and temporary chest pain (Doheny, 2021). This condition is more common in women who have recently experienced a traumatic life event like a health diagnosis, divorce, or the loss of a loved one.

Diabetes

It has been found that out of the total population of the U.S., 25% of those who are above the age of 65 years suffer from diabetes (Kirkman et al., 2012). As you probably know, when someone has diabetes, the concentration of glucose in their blood goes beyond the accepted normal level. This can cause damage to their kidneys, nerves, and eyes which can eventually lead to stroke or heart attack.

Moreover, as people age, they are more likely to develop conditions like high cholesterol and high blood pressure, which makes it even more difficult to keep diabetes under check.

Now, I know what you might be thinking: What does diabetes have to do with age? Well, as you age, your insulin resistance increases. Some of the factors responsible for this phenomenon are reduced physical activity, fat gain, and loss of mass or sarcopenia. And to top it all off, with age, the functioning power of the pancreas also decreases.

Dehydration

Since there is a huge change in body composition as people age, older adults are at a higher risk of developing dehydration. The feeling of becoming thirsty is your body's natural way of defending against dehydration. However, with age, this signal becomes less strong, and thus, people are not even able to realize when they need to drink water (WebMD Editorial Contributors, n.d.-a).

The total amount of body fluid starts decreasing with age, which is one of the reasons why older adults are at a higher risk of becoming dehydrated. Moreover, they lose a higher amount of water through urination because of reduced kidney function (Seladi-Schulman, 2020).

Adding to this is that older adults often fail to recognize the symptoms of dehydration while there's still time. Some of the initial signs include muscle cramps, dizziness, fatigue, and dry mouth. People who have problems related to cognitive impairment, like Alzheimer's, are also at a greater risk of dehydration since they may forget when they last drank water, and even if their body is telling them that it is thirsty, they may fail to identify those signals due to reduced cognitive ability.

Chronic Constipation

Almost everyone is going to experience constipation at some time or another in their lives, but when it comes to older adults, they are at a greater risk of experiencing it. Did you know that approximately one-third of the population of older adults go through constipation occasionally? (National Institute on Aging, n.d.). Some of the common causes of an increased rate of constipation in the elderly include not drinking and eating properly, dehydration, multiple chronic illnesses, and reduced mobility.

It has also been noticed that once people attain the age of 65 and above, the prevalence of constipation is greater in women than in men (Gallegos-Orozco et al., 2012). It was also found that 26% of women have a risk of developing chronic constipation compared to 16% of men. As they reach the age of 84, the percentage changes to 26% for men and 34% for women.

Conditions Related to Mental Health

According to known statistics, more than 20% of adults who are at least 60 years of age or more have a neurological or mental disorder (World Health Organization, 2017). The most common conditions that are diagnosed include mood disorders like bipolar disorder and depression, severe cognitive impairment, and anxiety. In fact, most of the suicide cases that are found are also because of mental health reasons. Approximately 5–7% of people who are above the age of 60 go through dementia and depression (WebMD Editorial Contributors, n.d.-b). Early diagnosis and prompt action is the key to treating mental disorders in older adults.

Fall Injuries

Fall injuries are extremely common among people above the age of 65. Even though it is considered inevitable, falls are something that you can prevent when sufficient steps are taken. In fact, did you know that one out of every four elderly persons in the United States falls every year? (Bergen et al., 2016). But the worst part is that less than 50% of the people who fall inform their doctor. (Stevens et al., 2012).

Moreover, out of all the hip fractures that older adults suffer from, more than 95% are because of a fall that happened sideways (Parkkari et al., 1999). Three-fourths of all hip fractures that take place are in women, with them suffering more fall injuries than men. With advancing age, fall injuries can be extremely serious because of the simple fact that the elderly might not ever recover from them.

At times, falls do not cause injury at all. But one out of every five falls' results in a grave injury like a head injury or a broken bone (Alexander et al., 2011). Sometimes, elderly who have already encountered a fall become so afraid that they develop a severe fear of falling even though they weren't injured the first time. Due to this fear, several older adults reduce their day-to-day activities, and when they are less active, it further enhances their chances of falling (Vellas et al., 1997).

Dementia

Did you know that approximately 40% of all dementia cases recorded every year can be either delayed or prevented? (Centers for Disease Control and Prevention, n.d.). Yes, which is why it is said that when we are talking about brain health, it's better that you have prior knowledge about what is normal and what isn't. When you age, your brain ages with you as well, which means that you will have more trouble multitasking, and your processing speed will become slower. However, there are some things that might improve with age, such as knowledge, skills, and routine memory. Forgetting certain things from time to time is considered normal, but when there is steady cognitive decline to the point that it is interfering with your day-to-day activities, it's best to consult an expert.

At present, almost 10 million new cases of dementia are registered every year, with more than 55 million people around the world suffering from this problem (World Health Organization, 2022). Approximately 60–70% of the cases of dementia that are recorded are Alzheimer's, which is the most common form. Depending on which part of the brain has been affected, the symptoms can differ from one person to another. Columbia University researchers have found that 22% of older adults above the age of 65 in the US suffer from mild cognitive impairment, whereas 10% of them have dementia (Manly et al., 2022).

Cardiovascular Disease

When people have reached the age of 65 or above, they are at a higher risk of developing cardiovascular diseases. Normal changes in the heart that happen with age include slight degeneration of the muscles, deposition of lipofuscin, also known as the aging pigment, thickening of the valves present inside the heart, and a heart murmur, which happens because of this change in valves (MedlinePlus, n.d.). Did you know that the most frequent reason for death in the elderly is due to cardiovascular disease? (Wei & Gersh, 1987). Yes, and not only that, but it is also a contributing factor to a significant number of disabilities that occur among the elderly.

For starters, the walls of the left ventricles in the heart become thick, irrespective of whether there is any change in blood pressure (Olivetti et al., 1991). The sinoatrial node has also been found to lose cells as people age. When compared to a person of 20 years of age, a person aged 75 has only 10% of the cells (Lye & Donnellan, 2000). The amount of blood the heart can hold also decreases because of the thickening of the heart walls, which, in turn, narrows down the chambers.

Bone and Joint Related Disorders

You have already learned about the various changes that happen to your bones and joints with age in the previous section of this chapter. Now, let's talk about arthritis—one of the common ailments in the elderly. According to recent statistics, one in every four adults in the United States suffers from arthritis that has been diagnosed by doctors (Barbour et al., 2017). Compared to men, this ailment is more prevalent among women. However, if they are involved in some kind of regular physical activity, then the symptoms can be managed, and it can also be a very good way to improve function and reduce pain.

Osteoporosis is another problem among the elderly. If you didn't know this already, your bone tissues are constantly broken down, and then new ones are built. But when you grow old, the rate of losing bone tissue becomes more than rebuilding new ones. Thus, the solid layer of bones starts to become thin and loses its strength. When the bone density reduces below a certain level, you develop osteoporosis. It is recommended that once you reach the age of 50 or if you break a bone around that age, you should get a bone density test done.

Now that you understand what changes your body is going through as you age, the next chapter focuses on strength training and how it can help manage or slow the effects of aging on your body.

2

WHY STRENGTH TRAIN?

 Strength does not come from physical capacity. It comes from an indomitable will.

— MAHATMA GANDHI

According to current research, strength training exercises can not only fight weakness and frailty but also the consequences that come with them. Performing regular exercise (for example, 2 to 3 days a week) can help you keep your bone density intact, build muscle strength, and gain independence and vitality with age (Seguin & Nelson, 2003). This chapter discusses the basics of strength training and its benefits for seniors. It also debunks strength training myths for seniors to help them stay motivated.

If you are a beginner, then you are probably unaware of the dos and don'ts of strength training, and it's crucial that you know them now; otherwise, you won't be able to reap the benefits. These tips will help you stay on the right path.

Let's start with the dos first.

- **Start with the right amount of weight.**

This is probably one of the first things that beginners are confused about. The best approach is to start with an amount that you won't have to fight to lift. You should be able to lift it comfortably a dozen times. If you are able to lift a weight at least 12 times and do three sets of this exercise, you will be able to build strong muscles. The weight you choose should be a balance between your comfort level and a range that slightly fatigues your muscles.

- **Focus on maintaining good form.**

Just like any other exercise, it's important that you perform the exercises correctly. This is because if you focus on your form, you are going to get good results in the long run. Moreover, when your form is incorrect, you are bound to experience pain in various parts of your body. If you see that maintaining form is becoming a challenge for you, you can start by decreasing the number of repetitions or the amount of weight (whichever is suitable for you). As a rule of thumb, always keep your feet shoulder-distance apart and your back straight, but if you are unsure about your form, consult a personal trainer.

- **Have a proper breathing pattern.**

Even if you are focusing on your form, one of the key aspects that get overlooked is your breathing pattern. And believe it or not, it plays a very important role. For starters, proper breathing ensures that your muscles are producing less carbon dioxide and that your workout efficiency is maximized (Davis, 2020). Secondly, it also helps in ensuring proper blood circulation. The one thing that you must keep in mind is that you should never hold your breath. As you are lifting the weight, breathe out, and when you are lowering the weight, breathe in.

- **Balance your training.**

It is important that you maintain a balanced approach while training your major muscle groups. This means that you must be mindful when you are scheduling your routine, keeping in mind that you must train both your lower and upper body muscles.

- **Make sure you have a rest day.**

Overtraining is a common mistake among beginners, and I don't want you to do the same. If you are training on consecutive days, avoid exercising the same set of muscles. You can choose to work on different sets of muscles on each day of the week, or you can mix and match your exercises in a way that you are working all your major muscles in a single session but maybe alternate days in a week.

Now, let's look at the common mistakes so that you have an idea about the don'ts.

- **Never skip stretching and warm-up.**

Many people seem to think that warm-ups are nothing but a waste of time, but that is not at all the case. If your muscles are cold, they will be more prone to incur injuries during the workout session. A simple 10-minute cardio session is often enough to start off your training and raise your body temperature, which helps your body throughout the rest of the session (Mayo Clinic Staff, 2021). When the temperature in your muscles rises, oxygen becomes more readily available to them; thus, they can relax and contract with ease, making it less challenging for you to perform strenuous exercises.

- **Don't rush during your reps.**

You have probably heard the saying, "slow and steady wins the race." This is applicable to strength training too. People seem to think that they can do more exercise in less time if they rush, but that's not how it works. The more you rush, the more your form will deteriorate, and you will not gain any benefit from your training and even experience muscle fatigue. But when you take it slow, you can focus on the muscle groups you want to train and can mindfully choose weights that you are comfortable with.

- **Don't overdo it.**

If you are training too much without giving your muscles sufficient time to rest in between, there is a high chance for you to suffer from injuries (Brumitt & Cuddeford, 2015). You must find the perfect balance between intensity and volume in order to maximize the benefit of strength training. Moreover, if you ever experience pain during your workouts, you should never ignore it. You should reduce the weight or take a few days off before resuming the session.

- **Don't wear the wrong shoes.**

Did you know that wearing the right type of shoes during strength training can reduce the chances of injury and speed up your progress? (Landsverk, 2021). Yes, and when you wear shoes catered to strength training, you will have better form and more stability.

So, I guess we are all now ready to learn more about strength training and how it can specifically benefit seniors.

WHAT'S STRENGTH TRAINING?

Were you of the opinion that workouts meant only cardio? Then it's time to rethink because there's much more to fitness than just that. I know that once you have reached the age of 60, it can be a little bit intimidating to think about lifting weights, but if you want a well-rounded approach to fitness and fight back frailty that comes with age, then including strength training in your training program is very important. But what is strength training really? It is a special type of exercise that involves lifting different weights and helps in building muscle strength. These exercises fall under the category of anaerobic exercise (Sundell, 2011). Some common forms of strength training include the usage of resistance bands, weight machines, and lifting free weights.

Types of Strength Training

Strength training is only a blanket term because there are seven different types that fall under it. If I ask you to conjure up an image in your mind of strength training, you will probably think of yourself lifting weights. That's completely natural because that's what most people perceive strength training to be. But once you learn about the different types, you will realize that you were probably doing these without even knowing that they are a part of strength training.

- **Agile strength:**

Agile strength is when you can change directions with power, precision, and strength, all of which start decreasing with increasing age. Seniors should especially work on agile strength because it will give them more independence. Moreover, you will be able to respond more quickly, which will prevent injuries and keep you safe—another important benefit of agile strength for seniors. This involves performing multi-directional workouts.

- **Endurance strength:**

As the term suggests, endurance strength is determined by your ability to go on for a longer period while carrying lighter loads. For seniors, several day-to-day activities require muscular endurance, such as carrying groceries or doing household chores. But indulging in moderate endurance exercises will help seniors overcome frailty and being easily fatigued. Here, you will be doing bodyweight workouts, and as you become stronger, you will be gradually adding more weight.

- **Explosive strength:**

It is with the help of explosive strength that you can move things with a lot of force. There is a misconception that explosive strength workouts are meant for athletes only but think of it like this: You have taken your grandson to the park, and they accidentally slipped from the top of a slide. You will have to exert all your strength suddenly to catch them in time. If you want such strength in your body, explosive strength training is what you need. Burpees, tuck jumps, and plyometric training are all examples of this type of strength training.

- **Maximum strength:**

This refers to the maximum weight a person can hold in a single rep, for example, in a deadlift or a bench press. It involves lifting heavy weights (as much as you are comfortable with) and doing ideally 1–4 reps with them.

- **Speed strength:**

This is about how fast a person can move. This type of training can be done by performing your reps at a faster rate, all while maintaining the right form or doing sprint workouts.

- **Starting strength:**

This is the movement you make in the beginning when there is no momentum, for example, the action of standing up from a chair. This type of strength training is important for improving your overall health and making your joints stronger. Sit-down squats and sprinter jumps are some great examples to incorporate for this type of training because it literally requires you to go from zero to sixty at once.

- **Relative strength:**

This type of training is exactly what its name suggests. It is a relative measure that analyzes your strength compared to your size. Relative strength cannot be improved by any specific type of exercise. Instead, you must focus on other types of strength training on this, and gradually, you will find your relative strength improving. To find your relative strength, divide the maximum number of reps you can do for a particular exercise by your body weight.

Things to Know and Consider When Doing Strength Training

Before you start strength training, here are some things you should know about it:

- **You don't have to be big in size to start strength training.**

Just because someone is big in size and has bigger muscles doesn't mean that they will have a better outcome or a better training experience. You could do just the same with smaller muscles.

- **Free weights work more muscles compared to machine weights.**

Many people are confused between free weights and machine weights when they are starting out. When you are using free weights, you must exercise the muscle groups other than the target group if you are willing to bring stability to your muscles during movement (Schott et al., 2019). On the contrary, when you are using machine weights, your movements will be largely restricted by the machinery's mechanism. In short, machine weights are great for beginners because they reduce the risk of injury and help to ensure the right form, but free weights are more beneficial in the long run as they help in functional fitness by helping you to work more muscles.

- **Eccentric exercises are more powerful but can also make you sore.**

Let me first explain to you what is meant by an eccentric movement and what is a concentric movement. Muscle contraction happens in a variety of ways and not just one. Imagine yourself walking up the stairs—this is an example of concentric contraction because here, the thigh muscles present at the front are shortening. However, eccentric contraction is when you are walking down the stairs, and the same muscles are lengthening. When compared, concentric contractions help burn more calories, but eccentric ones make you sore since they involve more muscle damage (Hody et al., 2019).

- **You can't expect to lose fat and increase muscle mass at the same time.**

Losing fat and gaining muscle mass are opposite metabolic processes, and your body is not wired to perform two such processes simultaneously. That is why it is advised that if you are following a weight loss regime, then you should work on maintaining a steady muscle mass (Cava et al., 2017).

Where to Start

Some people opt for a personal trainer, and some people don't. The choice is up to you. If you are worried that you don't have any equipment with you right now, and so you won't be able to start, don't worry because you don't really need any. Do you know why? There are certain exercises that you can try out, like planks and lunges, for which no external equipment is required; you simply need your own body weight.

Once you are comfortable with the idea of strength training, you can expand your schedule and include dumbbells. Another popular option to include is kettlebells. You could also include resistance bands once you are confident about your training program.

Whatever exercise you choose to do, it's best you start with 10–15 reps of each and then complete at least two sets. When you become comfortable, you can gradually increase the reps, the sets, and the weight.

How Hard or Intense Should the Workout Be for Seniors

There's no need for you to work out every day (contrary to popular belief) because, just like training, proper rest is equally crucial for your overall health and improvement. In fact, when you rest, that is when your muscles recover from the workout and grow. According to research, it is recommended that seniors should be performing strength training approximately two or three times a week (Fragala et al., 2019). But for high efficiency, you should be spreading out the exercises for different joints over the course of these few days.

When to Expect Results

Results will not have the same timeline for every person. Some might take months to see any changes, while others might see it in weeks. Your current fitness level is one of the determining factors as to when you will see the results, and in the same way, the makeup of your body also plays a role. Something that helps to achieve the results is having specific and clear goals in front of you so that you know exactly what you want. Sometimes people are not able to see results because the goals they have set for themselves are unrealistic for their body's abilities.

By now, you probably have a pretty good idea of what strength training is. Even if you are finding it difficult to lift weights now, keep in mind that things will get easier once you start gaining some muscle mass. So, be patient.

WHY DO YOU NEED STRENGTH TRAINING—12 REASONS

Strength training is one of the best ways to keep your muscles strong and healthy, even when you age. When you feel physically strong, it will automatically give a boost to your emotional well-being. But if you need to be more convinced, here are 12 reasons why strength training should be a part of your exercise regime as you age.

- **Reason #1—It boosts your metabolism.**

When you have a good metabolic rate, your body can burn calories at a much faster pace. But as you age, by way of nature, your metabolism slows down. That is why strength training becomes even more essential, as it helps in the development of muscle mass, which is metabolically better performing than fat. When your body's metabolic rate is high, it will reduce your chance of developing chronic illnesses, improve blood circulation, and ensure a steady reserve of energy throughout the day. Research has shown that strength training has the capability to enhance the metabolic rate by 72 hours post-exercise (Aristizabal et al., 2015).

- **Reason #2—It helps strengthen your body and build muscle mass.**

Even though it's true that you realistically cannot stop the aging process, you can take measures to deal with the symptoms. One such measure is incorporating strength training. Studies have revealed that approximately 30% of elderly people who are over the age of 70 face problems with day-to-day activities like climbing stairs, getting up from a chair, and walking (Freedman & Martin, 1998). Apart from that, whenever you start encountering limitations to your mobility, it will lead to higher rates of mortality, nursing home admission, chronic disease, and falls. But if someone can maintain an active lifestyle and incorporate strength training into their schedule, this average decline of power and strength can be kept in check.

- **Reason #3—It helps to burn fat.**

If you didn't know this already, strength training also helps in reducing fat mass since it helps in building lean muscles. When you age, you tend to gain more fat (especially women). More fat also means that you have a higher risk of developing certain chronic illnesses. But research has shown that strength training alone can help reduce 1.4% of your total body fat, which is almost similar to what aerobics or cardio can do (Wewege et al., 2021).

- **Reason #4—It counteracts the reduction in bone density.**

Reduced bone density with age means that you become more prone to fractures. There have been numerous studies so far that found that strength training can actually slow down the rate of bone loss and also help in building new bone cells (Harvard Health Publishing, 2021). Wondering how this happens? Well, when you perform activities that put pressure on your bones, it can give a slight nudge to the inactive bone-forming cells.

- **Reason #5—It helps reduce bone porosity.**

Since the bone density increases, the bone porosity decreases, automatically making your bones stronger, and you no longer need to worry about major fractures from minor falls.

- **Reason #6—It eases stiffness in joints.**

With age, if you think about swimming (even a few laps) or a short walk around the block, it can seem excessively painful. This is because the joints become stiff. Strength training has been found to reduce stiffness and pain by 35% in seniors and enhance the functioning of lower limbs by 33% (Latham & Liu, 2010).

- **Reason #7—It can improve your reflexes and reaction times.**

Up until now, you have only learned about the physical benefits of strength training. Did you know that it can positively influence your nervous system as well? When you exercise, more blood starts flowing into your brain, which reduces your reaction time and boosts your reflexes (Lord & Castell, 1994).

- **Reason #8—It improves your aerobic capacity.**

Aerobic capacity is the maximum amount of oxygen a person can utilize per unit of body weight and time. The effects of strength training on increasing the aerobic capacity of the elderly have been proven by research (Frank et al., 2015).

- **Reason #9—It helps you stay independent.**

As you age, you probably want to do all your chores by yourself and not depend on others, but this becomes next to impossible because of mobility issues. According to past research, strength training is known to help with posture, coordination, and balance (Cadore et al., 2013). When your balance improves, you can take care of yourself, do basic chores without another person's help, and be more independent.

- **Reason #10—It reduces fall risk.**

Even though it's true that you might not be able to prevent a fall completely, strength training can reduce the chances in seniors.

After reaching a certain age, you might feel unsteady, even while doing basic things like getting up from a chair or bending down to pick up something, which increases your risk of falling. But a combination of balance and strength training for seniors is the perfect approach to reduce the chances of fractures and falls (Zouita et al., 2020).

- **Reason #11—It strengthens the immune system.**

There have been several studies over the past decade that have demonstrated the role of strength training in fortifying the immune system. A scientific review published in 2019 has already studied the connection between regular physical activity and improvement in immune response (Nieman & Wentz, 2019). It stated that since there is an increase in the flow of blood throughout the body when you exercise, it subsequently leads to increased circulation of immune cells as well, specifically T cells and natural killer cells that are responsible for wiping out the pathogens from your body.

- **Reason #12—It has a positive impact on mental health.**

There are several ways in which strength training can benefit the elderly with respect to their mental health. When you lift weights, it releases feel-good hormones in your body, also known as endorphins, that lift your mood and keep you happy (American Psychological Association, 2020). It has also been linked with eliminating depressive symptoms in the elderly (Gordon et al., 2018). Regularly engaging in strength training also reduces levels of cortisol (stress hormone) in the body, lessening bouts of anxiety and stress (Gordon et al., 2020).

By now, you must have realized that strength training has clear benefits for all parts of your body. Now, let us debunk some common myths to have a better understanding of this form of physical workout.

DON'T BELIEVE THESE!

It's important to debunk some of the common misconceptions about strength training for seniors so that you no longer feel overwhelmed by them.

- **I'm too old for strength training.**

Whether you are 20 or 60, you are never too late to start strength training. In fact, research has proven that strength training is beneficial to seniors to such an extent that it should be recommended by general physicians, too (Travers et al., 2019). To play it safe, it's advisable that you start by incorporating strength training into your routine only twice a week and then work your way up from there.

- **I cannot strength train because of my bad [insert body part].**

It's true that injuries can be frustrating and can create additional hurdles along the way, but they will never completely stop you from strength training. All you need is a dedicated program suited to your needs, keeping in mind your level of flexibility and joint health. Let's say your shoulder is your weak point. You can still strength train the rest of your body without putting strain on your shoulder.

- **Strength training will make me bulky.**

This is a very common misconception among women that strength training is going to make them look bulky. A bulkier physique is a result of fat accumulation, and in strength training, you burn fat and gain muscles which, in fact, will help you acquire a leaner appearance.

- **Elderly people cannot gain muscles.**

I have seen many seniors back down from strength training just because they think this will not bring them any result whatsoever in terms of muscle mass. But according to research, high-intensity strength training can increase body strength in seniors (Evans, 1999). You also need to incorporate exercises into your regime that involve more than one joint and muscle group at a time.

- **It is only meant for men.**

If you think that strength training is only meant for men, it's time you see things from a different perspective because the days when only men dominated the gym are over. Did you know that in 2015, more than 87,000 women took part in the

CrossFit Games Open, and more than 25% were above the age of 40? (Sole-Smith, 2015).

- **I will become less flexible with strength training.**

As outrageous as it may sound, some people believe that they will lose their flexibility if they engage in strength training. But it's exactly the opposite that happens. When you strength train, you gain better mobility as you exercise the full range of motion in all your joints, which also helps in muscle flexibility.

- **Strength training is not safe.**

Regardless of whether you are strength training or not, when you age, there is a risk of injury in almost everything you do, so you must be careful. So, when you are lifting weights, you need to have proper knowledge about how things should be done, how you must maintain your posture and form, and what safety procedures should be followed. Don't push yourself too hard on the repetitions and work your way up the ladder slowly. Skilled physiotherapists have always supported the idea of incorporating strength training in the daily exercise routine of seniors so that they can perform their day-to-day activities with more confidence and ease.

ACHIEVE A STRONG BODY WITH THESE TIPS

Everyone wants to lead a happy life, but with age, we are all attacked by frailty and mobility issues, making us more dependent on others and hitting our self-esteem. If you don't want the same thing happening to you, strength training is the way out. In this section, we will explore some expert tips on strength training that will not only help you get started but also ensure that your training is effective and safe.

- **Add strength training to your routine at least twice a week.**

Is your definition of a workout something like going for a run around the block? Well, that's the case with most older people because they think cardio is all they can do. But they are missing out on all the fun by skipping strength training. If you are one of them too, and you have been skipping strength training because of all the negative thoughts in your mind (such as "What would people say?" or "Is strength training safe?"), it's time you remove your mental barriers. Research says that including strength training in your routine for a minimum of two days a week can help muscle growth (Schoenfeld et al., 2016).

- **Plan your warm-up and cool-down.**

When you start a new exercise regime, all you can probably think of is jumping straight into the action, but that's exactly what you shouldn't be doing. Every workout should precede a warm-up session and end with a proper cool-down session. When you warm up, it gets your heart beating faster and pumps more blood to all your muscles. When you are starting out, do a gentle warm-up like swinging your arms or walking in place, and then you can increase the pace by doing a few jumping jacks or other range-of-motion workouts. Similarly, for the cool-down sequence, perform some stretching exercises that will prevent muscle cramping. Try to hold each posture for about 10 to 20 seconds. Your flexibility will improve if you are able to hold for longer but don't push yourself too much.

- **Be easy on your joints.**

Your hip and your knee are two of the most complex joints present in your body, bearing a lot of weight and having many tiny structures within them. So, when you are starting out, be careful about the amount of weight you are putting on them. Start with small amounts that you can comfortably take, and once you become habituated, you can increase the weight, reps, or both. This is even more important if you have joint issues.

- **Start with exercises that rely on your body weight.**

Strength training is not only about lifting weights. Yes, you heard that right! There are also exercises that can be done simply with the help of your own body weight. In fact, lifting your own weight is something you should be comfortable with before you start lifting excess weights. You can perform exercises like push-ups, squats, lunges, plank, and jumping jacks.

- **Set realistic goals.**

When you step into a strength training program for the first time and learn about all it can do for you, it can be tempting to set high and mighty goals. But think about what you can realistically achieve.

WHERE'S THE MOTIVATION?—OVERCOME THE BARRIERS

I understand that it is not always easy to muster up the motivation to work out on a regular basis or to overcome the barriers in front of you, especially when you have a ton of other things on your to-do list. While everyone is aware of the positive impact of exercise, sometimes the benefits alone are not enough to push you off your couch. So, here are some tips to stay motivated.

- **Change your routine to make it fun.**

You will find that there are people who like to start off their exercise schedule by walking on a treadmill at the gym. On the contrary, there are others who find this same activity bland. What might seem fun to you might not be the same to someone else. So, be creative and change your routine from time to time. If you are feeling a little burned out on strength training, take a day off and go on an adventure. Revive your soul and resume. You can also mix up strength training with weekly Zumba classes. Remember that consistency is key. As long as you are involved in some form of physical activity daily and enjoy yourself, everything is good.

- **Make it social.**

When you make your workout social, that is, if you work out with a friend, you have an accountability partner. This not only gives you a mental boost, but that person is there to pull you up even on days when you don't feel like working out. If, someday, you are not able to hit the gym because of traffic or bad weather, you can get your friend on a video call and work out together. It's better than breaking the streak. If you can't find common friends, you can try Zumba classes or dance classes.

- **Keep track of your progress.**

Logging your workouts is essential to understand how far you have come. This also helps motivate you when you feel you haven't progressed at all. Moreover, when you are keeping track of your workouts, you are more likely to reach your goals. Maintain a workout journal where you will be jotting down the exercises you have done each week, the number of reps, and the amount of weight you have lifted. Also, make it a point to write a little bit about how that exercise schedule made you feel.

- **Set sustainable goals.**

If you have not been exercising at all, setting a goal of exercising two hours every day might be too much to expect. A better approach would be to start incorporating smaller steps. For example, take the stairs instead of an elevator, walk to the grocery store around the block, park at the furthest spot in malls and walk the rest of the way, and so on. Once you become a little bit habituated to the increase in physical activity, you can start by incorporating 20 minutes of physical workout every day. In the beginning, start with movements you enjoy and then progress gradually.

- **Envision a healthier, happier you.**

We might not realize it, but sometimes the negative thoughts that reside in our subconscious mind are more powerful than we know. It is essential that you utilize the power of visualization and envision yourself as a healthier and happier person. Remember that you are not striving for perfection but progress. So, leave your self-criticism behind and work toward the goals you have set for yourself.

- **Make the right use of technology.**

Seniors are often overwhelmed when it comes to learning new tech, but at the same time, there are a growing number of people out there who have incorporated technology into their training programs and couldn't be more grateful for their decision. For example, you can start using pedometers. Research has shown that people who were previously leading a sedentary lifestyle were able to increase their daily activity by approximately 2000 steps by wearing a pedometer (Mansi et al., 2014).

- **Encourage the feeling of usefulness.**

When you approach old age, you increasingly feel that you are no longer useful to anyone in any way. That feeling alone is enough to make you feel unmotivated to do stuff. That is why it is essential to keep the feeling of usefulness alive. Attend events at your locality where you can do some volunteering work over the weekends. This is one of the best ways to socialize and make you feel that what you do is valuable to society.

- **Find accountability.**

Sometimes a little bit of support can do wonders for your fitness routine. That is why it is advised that you start working out with a partner. It can be a friend or even someone from your family. It will be a habit to always show up for the workout when you know that someone else is counting on you. If you found it hard to hit the gym earlier, now it will no longer be about you. In fact, a study has found that 95% of the people who started a specific program with someone they knew were able to see it through to the end (Wing & Jeffery, 1999).

- **Seek help from a professional.**

If all other steps don't seem to be working out for you, maybe what you need is a personal trainer. A very common reason among seniors for not feeling motivated is when they are working out but not seeing the results they want. This is usually because they are not performing the exercises correctly. This is where a professional can help you by evaluating your program and goals and making the necessary tweaks. Sometimes, when you are all by yourself, it is much easier to slack off. But when you have a trainer, they will cheer you on and help set weekly goals.

- **Eliminate barriers.**

Sometimes it's the mental barriers that are keeping us from exercising, and these barriers are not set up by someone else; we internalize them subconsciously. One such barrier is fear. Starting a new workout regime can be scary (more so for someone who hasn't ever tried it before), and sometimes you might feel like skipping the ordeal rather than making yourself look like an idiot. Another mental barrier is frustration. Progress is gradual, but it is also very slow, and people are not always patient. So, they might get frustrated and quit before seeing any real progress. There are several other mental barriers like this, for example, boredom, confusion, and dislike for exercise.

- **Eliminate excuses.**

I'm pretty sure all of you have used excuses in your life at least once to escape a situation. Using excuses to escape exercise is very common. One very common excuse is, "I don't have enough time." For starters, if you are doing a 30-minute workout session, it is taking up only 2% of your day. So, do you still want to say you don't have time? Next, I often hear seniors complaining, "I'm too tired." Well, the best thing about strength training is that it can make you feel more energized. But if you do feel too tired to work out, it's high time you revisit your sleeping schedule. Eating food items rich in magnesium can also give you a boost of energy. Whatever your excuses are, remember that you can achieve anything you want if you decide you are going to do it with all your willpower.

Now that you have a deeper understanding of strength training and how it can help you become stronger as you age, the next chapter focuses on getting started with the exercises.

Disclaimer: This book does not provide medical advice. The content of this book is provided for reference and education purposes only. The information presented here should not be used to make a diagnosis or to replace or overrule a qualified healthcare provider's judgment. The exercises and workouts described in this book may not be suitable for everyone, and it is essential to consult a physician before starting any new exercise routine.

The author and publisher of this eBook are not liable for any injuries, damages, or losses that may result from performing the exercises and workouts described in this eBook. The user assumes all risks and responsibilities associated with performing any exercise or workout described in this eBook.

The information in this eBook is based on the author's research and experience in the field of strength training. However, individual results may vary, and the author cannot guarantee the accuracy, completeness, or efficacy of the information in this eBook.

By downloading and using this eBook, the user acknowledges that they have read and understood this disclaimer and agree to use the information in this eBook at their own risk.

3

KICKSTART YOUR JOURNEY

This chapter helps you start your strength training journey by shedding light on what you need to begin the journey. It will also discuss seniors' safety guidelines, including warm-ups, cool-downs, reps, and sets.

If you still think that strength training is not a good remedy for people with osteoporosis, let me tell you the success story of Betty, who was diagnosed with severe osteoporosis but is now much better after following a regular strength training program. She had mostly been in a sedentary lifestyle, doing a desk job and coming back home without engaging in any form of workout whatsoever. She was 63 when she started strength training, and six months in, she started noticing significant changes to her bone density. This could happen to you too. If you are worried about how you will be starting this journey, don't worry, I will be covering all the basics in this chapter.

START WITH THE EQUIPMENT

Studies have revealed that approximately 67% of older adults have remained sedentary for more than 8.5 hours every day (Harvey et al., 2013). Even though you might want to spend your senior years having quality time with your grandkids or catching up on all the books you weren't able to read, it's important that you also find the time to include some workouts, especially strength training. If finding the right equipment is something you are confused about, there are a lot of affordable equipment for seniors out there that you can use to start your journey to becoming stronger. However, you must keep in mind that the type of equipment you use also depends on the type of strength training exercise you want to include in your program.

Resistance Bands

These are one of the best pieces of equipment you can buy when you don't want to spend too much and yet want to get a taste of strength training. These are lightweight tubes or ropes that can be stretched and are comparatively easier to handle than free weights, especially for an elderly person who is just starting out. Resistance bands are available in all different sizes and shapes, and you can wrap them around your arms and legs, which makes movements even more difficult and thus assists in engaging more muscles in your body. One of the benefits of resistance bands is that they don't apply too much force on the joints but rather on the muscles, so if you have issues with joint pain, you can safely use it without any risk of injury.

In today's world, people are so habituated to sitting at their desks and slouching over their laptops and computers that it leads to what is known as forward head posture and slouched shoulders. A recent study found that this type of posture can lead to reduced spine mobility, which can further negatively affect respiratory functioning and lead to a higher risk of death among the elderly (Blum, 2019). However, if they can implement resistance bands in their exercise regime, it can strengthen the abdominal and back muscles and counteract the damage caused to the spine and reduce the stress on that particular area.

In a meta-analysis, it was stated that resistance bands could enhance balance and flexibility in seniors, which in turn can reduce the risk of falls and accidents in them (Yeun, 2017).

Light Weights

If you thought that you only had to lift heavy weights to get good results from your strength training program, then you were wrong. In fact, seniors who are just starting out and have some extra space in their homes should get light weights because they will help you sustain your program in the long run and prevent any injuries. Researchers at McMaster University concluded that whether you are using light weights or heavy weights for strength training, there would not be any significant difference in the result you achieve as long as you are growing tired at the end of the session (Reynolds, 2016). So, in simpler words, it is the effort that you are putting into the workout that matters. As a beginner, if you jump towards lifting heavier weights, you will tend to have a poorer range of motion, which will not benefit you in any way. On the other hand, light weights will help you achieve a full range of motion. A study published in the *Journal of Strength and Conditioning Research* stated that when people performed strength training with a full range of motion, they witnessed more growth in the size of their muscles (McMahon et al., 2014).

Good Walking/Training Shoes

As you all know by now, one of the most important things about strength training is maintaining proper form; shoes are very important for that. Research shows that wearing good training shoes during workouts can prevent injuries (Nigg et al., 2015).

However, the type of shoes you are supposed to buy usually depends on the type of workout you are going to do. For example, running shoes have sufficient arch support and midsole cushioning, whereas strength training shoes usually have elevated heels. The heel height you choose for your shoes should be something you are comfortable with, even while doing a squat, and, at the same time, doesn't hamper your ability to maintain an upright posture.

Chair for Seated Exercises

Seated exercises are considered very good for seniors, especially because they do not put much pressure on the joints while reducing the risk of injuries. When people age, it's natural for them to spend most of their time seated—a factor that deteriorates their posture even more. This is where chair exercises come in. They can support the spine and strengthen the shoulders. Stretching your muscles through various seated exercises also enhances stability in the elderly.

As people age, blood flow to different parts of the body reduces, which causes tingling and numbness in their legs and arms. But chair exercises can get the blood flowing to the farthest parts of the body, thus relieving the elderly of this discomfort. Before you buy the chair, keep in mind that the chair should be ergonomic with respect to your height and the type of poses you want to practice.

Wrist Weights

If you don't want to increase the duration of your workout but want to take it up a notch, that is when wrist weights come to the rescue. You can wear them when you are going out for a run or during your strength training workout. The first and foremost benefit of these wearable weights is their role in supporting weight loss, which has been proven by research (Ohlsson et al., 2020). The next benefit is that they are very easy to use and thus perfect for beginners. Moreover, you don't need to enroll in any complicated program to be able to use them or have an elaborate space to train with them. You can simply take a walk, in a nearby park. If you have arthritis or some other kind of degenerative joint disease, then it's quite natural for you to find it difficult to hold weights in your hands. In that case, wearing wrist weights is a great option.

Wrist weights are usually available in the range of 1 to 10 pounds.

Yoga Mat

Yoga mats are preferred by people of all ages, and for good reason. Ever since they came into existence, they have been a hit among fitness freaks. For seniors, it is advised that you get anti-slip yoga mats so that you can get a better grip and stay safe from all kinds of falls. One of the prime factors to consider before buying a yoga mat is comfort. If you want to be sure that nothing will happen to your joints, you can get mats that provide an additional layer of cushioning. Another factor to keep in mind is the size of the mat. It should be appropriate with respect to your body.

Stability Ball

Stability balls are a very good piece of equipment for people willing to focus on their fitness. They not only enhance your core strength and muscle tone but also work towards improving your balance. Experts often recommend using stability balls during your stretching and warm-up exercises, for example, while doing sit-ups and crunches, because this will help to expand your range of motion. When you learn to use the stability ball correctly, it can help to strengthen your lower back and abdominal muscles. These are the muscles that you use for performing your day-to-day activities, and so when you train them, you can do your daily chores all by yourself, without any external help. Leg lifts and hip circles are some common exercises that seniors perform with the help of a stability ball.

Dumbbells

Irrespective of your age, dumbbells are always going to be one of the best ways for you to work out and train your muscles. Having dumbbells at home also makes it easier for you not to miss a workout on days when you don't want to go to the gym. It's advisable that you keep at least three different weights of dumbbells so that you can perform different types of workouts and, depending on the strength of your muscles, shuffle between the weights you use for each type of exercise. The most common question that people have in their mind is what weight they should be using while starting out. Well, the weight that you choose should be heavy enough for you to perform approximately 12 reps, but not comfortably. By the time you reach the 10th rep, your muscles should be tiring out, and you should be struggling to do those last two reps. If this happens to you, you'll know that you have chosen the right amount of weight for your exercise.

Kettlebells

Kettlebells are extremely convenient to handle. It's true that they might require a little bit of space to practice, but other than that, they will improve your grip, enhance bone density, and help you work on your confidence levels too. Kettlebells are the perfect mélange of high-intensity cardio and weight training, making them perfect for seniors. The kettlebell swings are also popular for helping you improve your posture. The back portion of your body consists of a special set of muscles known as posterior chain muscles. According to research, when your posterior chain muscles are strong, it reduces the risk of injuries, improves athletic performance, improves posture, and alleviates back pain (De Ridder et al., 2013). And do you know what? Kettlebell swings are one of the best exercises you can do to improve and strengthen your posterior chain muscles.

So, now that you have a better idea about the equipment to use, we will move on to the next most important aspect of workouts —your workout outfit.

WHAT SHOULD I WEAR?

Did you know that research has shown that there is a direct connection between your performance levels during workouts and what you wear? (March, 2018). Moreover, most of the injuries that happen to people during exercising are because they don't have the right kind of equipment or activewear. The type of clothing you choose should be high-quality compression wear. The main reason behind this is that these types of clothing increase the flow of blood to the heart and maintain proper circulation. When you are working out, your muscles always need a steady supply of oxygen, and good blood circulation will ensure that. It will also help reduce soreness and fatigue by controlling the accumulation of lactic acid.

A survey performed on 2,000 gym goers concluded that 69% of them preferred going to the gym when they had nice workout clothing on because it acted as an added motivation (Schmall,

2021). When you love what you see in the mirror before working out, it automatically creates a positive mindset, which is extremely important for you to stay on your path and not get distracted or give up because of the lack of progress. The color of your activewear also plays a role. Choose colors that make you feel energetic. According to research, athletes often prefer red-colored clothing because it makes them feel dominant (Elliot, 2015). However, the association with color might not be universal. You might relate to a different color altogether. So, if it's green that lifts your spirits, buy something in green.

Now, let us be a bit more specific. Since we are talking about strength training for seniors, there are certain aspects of activewear that must be kept in mind. In general, they should be perfectly sized and comfortable, but if you want a detailed breakdown of the things to look out for while choosing activewear for strength training, here you go.

- **Choose spandex if you are into Pilates.**

Pilates is something that will require you to perform a lot of stretching and bending, and spandex is the material that comes to mind when you talk about flexibility.

- **Avoid fabrics that are not breathable.**

Irrespective of the type of workout you do, one thing is for sure: You will be sweating a lot, and if you wear a fabric that is not breathable, it will be highly uncomfortable, as it will not allow your body heat to pass through. That is why experts often advise going for wicking fabrics, which are mainly synthetic fabrics that "wick" the sweat away and thus allow your body to cool down.

- **Choose the right fit.**

The fit of your clothes is another important factor to keep in mind. They shouldn't be uncomfortable, for starters. At the same time, if you are thinking about cycling or running, make sure you don't wear wide-legged pants, as they can increase the chances of accidents. In simpler terms, your clothes should be comfortable but shouldn't get in the way of your workouts.

- **Adjust your clothes with the seasons.**

This is a point people often overlook. During the summer months, you must choose clothes that will keep you cool and take away your sweat. Similarly, during the winter months, you need to dress in layers to stay protected from the cold, especially if you are planning on working out in the open.

- **Sports bras shouldn't dig into your skin.**

Choosing the right sports bra is a whole ordeal. According to research, buying the right type of sports bra can lessen discomfort and breast pain during workouts (Mason et al., 1999). If you choose an ill-fitted sports bra that digs into your skin, the first problem that you will experience is chaffing around your shoulders. So, you need to first consider the type of activities you are going to do. For example, yoga is a low-impact activity, whereas running is a high-impact one. In general, a more supportive sports bra is required when you are engaging in high-impact workouts (Norris et al., 2021). The next thing to consider is the cup design. There are basic types to choose from: encapsulation sports bras (required during intense activities), compression sports bras (for low-impact activities), and combination sports bras (for a variety of activities).

YOUR RULEBOOK TO SAFETY

Strength training is a safe form of working out when you follow the general rules and guidelines that are present. I am proud that you have finally made the decision to be active and have taken the initial steps to chart out a workout program for yourself, but the next step is to know about the safety rules in place so that you don't end up hurting yourself in the process. But before we move on to the preventive measures, I want to discuss some of the common injuries that can result if you are not careful so that you are more aware.

Injuries From Strength Training

I know that you already have enough reasons in your mind that are keeping you from working out, so this section is not meant to scare you but to educate you about the injuries that might occur if you are not wary about the technique and form while doing strength training.

- **Rotator cuff injuries:**

The muscles present around your shoulders are termed rotator cuff muscles. Sometimes, strength training can lead to shoulder pain due to a tear in these muscles. If this happens to you, you will find it challenging to do even the most basic tasks in your day-to-day life, like brushing your teeth or lifting a chair. There are two types of rotator cuff injuries that mostly happen to people: tendinopathy and rotator cuff tear. The former happens around the tendons of your rotator cuff muscles when they are unable to repair themselves, whereas the latter happens after you have dislocated your shoulder, had a traumatic injury or excess wear and tear from degenerative disease.

- **Hamstring pulls:**

If you've ever had a hamstring pull (I really hope you don't have to go through it), you'll know it instantly. It appears like a sharp and shooting pain that goes up the back of your thigh. If you have been doing a lot of powerful movements like sprinting or jumping, it can put pressure on your hamstring muscles, which can cause a tear. Sometimes they can heal within a short period of time, but if the injury is serious, it can take an entire year.

- **Tennis elbow:**

This is a common injury caused by over-gripping. If you have repeatedly been moving your arms and wrists, it can lead to this injury, and the most common symptom is pain around the outside portion of your elbow. This injury often occurs due to poor technique, which is why I often reinforce the importance of good form and technique during strength training.

- **Disc herniations:**

When you have poor lifting techniques, it is highly likely for you to encounter disc herniations, which is basically a type of back injury. If you have been experiencing a tingling feeling down your back that goes all the way down to the legs and numbness in your lower back region, it's possible that you have a herniated disc. Each vertebral bone in your body is separated by vertebral discs that help in cushioning. But due to repetitive poor movement, these discs can rupture, resulting in this type of injury.

- **Tendonitis:**

Tendonitis occurs when you develop tears in the tendons of your body, which makes it difficult to have smooth motion because of the inflammation in the tendons. The area where tendonitis has occurred might become red and even swell.

- **Back strain:**

Overstretching and heavy lifting with incorrect form often result in muscle spasms and tears, causing stiffness and back strain.

- **Biceps strain:**

Micro tearing of the biceps is rare, but when it happens, it can lead to biceps strain or biceps tendonitis. This can happe once again, due to poor technique or even due to overuse.

Prevent Injuries

Whether you are trying out strength training to combat sarcopenia or simply to stay active, the one thing that you don't want is to get hurt, so here are some tips you should follow.

- **Never miss your warm-up and cool-down sessions.**

This will not only help to loosen up your muscles but also get the blood flowing.

- **Don't push yourself beyond what's comfortable.**

If you can't control a weight, it automatically increases your chances of injury. So, never let people push you into lifting weights that you can't handle.

- **Build up slowly.**

Even when you have learned the technique and you have mastered the form, if you increase the weight too fast, you risk an injury. Take things slowly. It is often advised that you should increase the weight only when you feel that you would be able to do one more rep without any kind of cheating.

- **Take breaks.**

Did you know that overtraining can slow down your progress? That is why it is recommended that you take regular breaks in between, and you should not train if you are feeling ill or overtired.

- **Ask for help if you need it rather than struggling.**

If you are trying out a new exercise, a new form, or maybe lifting a heavier weight, it might be that you are not feeling too confident about it. That's completely natural, and there's nothing to feel shy about. Rather than struggling with your workout and doing it the wrong way, why not do it with a partner? You can also ask for the help of a qualified personal trainer or a gym instructor who can guide you the right way. Whatever you decide to do, just don't let your ego get in the way and keep you from asking for help.

- **Wear the correct gear.**

We have already established the importance of wearing the correct gear in this chapter. When you dress appropriately and comfortably, they allow you to sweat easily, and most importantly, they do not restrict your movements.

- **Fuel yourself correctly.**

If you continue to train diligently but don't pay attention to your nutrition, it will impact your overall health. So, it's important that you maintain a nutritious diet along with workouts that will keep you energized.

- **Learn proper technique.**

People encounter injuries because of incorrect technique, which makes it very crucial for you to understand the technique before you jump into a workout program.

- **Listen to your body.**

Your body needs time to repair itself after you have worked out. So, it's better for seniors to leave a day's gap between workouts, especially when starting out. And, if you are not feeling well someday, don't force yourself. Get some rest and start the next day.

WHY STRETCH BEFORE AND AFTER YOUR WORKOUT?

What comes to your mind when you think about stretching? Do you think that it's only for gymnasts and dancers? Well, guess what? There are many benefits to stretching, especially when you do it before and after your workout. When you stretch on a regular basis, it keeps your muscles healthy and more flexible—both of which keep chronic muscle pain at bay. Let's explore the plus points of stretching in greater detail.

Before a Workout

There are some very specific advantages of stretching before you start a workout. You don't have to do it for too long. Spending 5 to 10 minutes is sufficient to reap these benefits.

1. The first thing it does is improve circulation and blood flow to every muscle of your body (Hotta et al., 2013). Now, if you are wondering how this is beneficial to you in terms of your workout program, well, because of the increased blood flow, you experience reduced muscle soreness and a shortened recovery period.
2. Secondly, when you stretch regularly, it helps in improving your flexibility. This will give you a greater range of motion, and you will find it easier to perform the workout.
3. Finally, research has shown that stretching prepares your muscles for all types of workouts (Opplert & Babault, 2017). Because of the two benefits mentioned above, it results in enhanced overall performance.

After a Workout

Once your workout is over, I'm sure you might feel like running straight into the shower, but that's exactly what you shouldn't be doing. In fact, you shouldn't sit to scroll through your Facebook either! What you should be doing instead (yes, you probably guessed it already) is stretching for another 5 to 10 minutes.

The benefits of post-workout stretch:

1. When you stretch after your workout, it reduces your chances of injury and muscle strains.
2. Stretching after workouts paves the way for gradual relaxation. This is not only great for your body but for your mind too.
3. When you work out, your body produces a lot of lactic acids, which make you feel tired and achy after the session. However, stretching can reduce the amount of lactic acid in your body and prevent these issues.

WARMING UP AND COOLING DOWN

You already learned the importance of warming up and cooling down, and now it's time you learn how to do these two things through stretching exercises. For your ease of understanding, I have divided this section into three parts. So, we will be looking into stretching exercises for the chest, shoulders, and arms.

Chest

Even though all of you have different levels of flexibility, these stretching exercises will help you work on your muscles and improve your range of motion with time.

Behind-the-Back Elbow-to-Elbow Grip

This is one of the best stretching exercises that you can perform, not only before and after your workouts but also anytime during the day.

- Start in a standing or seated position. Your hands should be at your sides—hanging down—and your shoulders should be straight and pressed downwards.
- Broaden your chest gently by squeezing your shoulder blades together.
- Slowly bring one arm behind your back and then the other. Then, grip elbow to elbow.

Above-the-Head Stretch

This stretching exercise can also be performed in the standing and seated positions.

- Start by interlocking your fingers. Slowly bend your elbows and then raise both your arms. Take a deep breath while you lift your arms behind your head.
- Squeeze your shoulders gently. Meanwhile, try to push your hands and neck a little backward to maintain the tension.
- Hold this position for about half a minute and then release.

Bent-Arm Wall Stretch

- Stand near a wall with a straight posture. Your right arm should be kept on the wall at a 90-degree angle.
- Press your bicep, forearm, and palm on the wall entirely.

- Now, turn your body slowly towards your left to intensify the effect of the stretch, and hold this position for about 30 seconds before you switch your arms.

Extended Child's Pose

- Start by sitting on your heels.
- Your knees should be hip width apart. Bring your head down very slowly until it touches the floor.
- Bring your arms in front of you and stretch them comfortably. For an even better stretch, press your palms on the floor and try to touch your forehead to the surface as well.
- Hold this position for about 20 seconds and take a few deep breaths.
- When you rise, inhale.

Side Lying Parallel Arm Chest Stretch

- Start by lying face down on the floor. Slowly bring both your arms to the sides so that your body resembles the shape of the letter "T," and make sure your palms are facing the floor.
- Now, slowly apply pressure on your left hand and roll towards your right side. Lift your left leg gently and bend it. To gain more stability in this position, place your left foot behind you, just at the back of your extended right leg.
- Stay in this position for about half a minute and then repeat the steps on the other side.

- If you want to deepen the effect of this stretch, you can also try to raise the opposite hand upwards (towards the ceiling).

Shoulders

Whether you want to keep injuries at bay or you are experiencing pain in the shoulder region, these stretching exercises can be extremely handy.

Shoulder Rolls

Shoulder rolls are known to release the tension at the back of your neck and shoulder region and are especially good if you have been feeling a little hunchback lately.

- You can do this exercise both in a standing and sitting position. Ensure that you have a neutral spine and keep your shoulders down. Squeeze your shoulders back as much as you can.
- Keep your arms at your sides and slowly move your shoulders in a circular pattern, bringing them up and backward. Your torso should not be moving.
- Perform the rolls in this manner 10 times. Once done, repeat the same thing in a forward direction another 10 times.

Shoulder Press-Ups

The shoulder press-up is a variation of the normal press-up or push-up that enhances stability and strength in the triceps and shoulders.

- Take the position of a normal push-up, but the difference is that your hands should be a little bit more than shoulder-distance apart. Keep your elbows locked in position, your toes on the ground, and your hips toward the ceiling. Your posture should look like a "V," only in an upside-down fashion.
- Then, slowly bring the top of your head down toward the ground. Don't allow your head to contact the floor. Just before contact, pause and return to the starting position.
- Make sure you keep your shoulders locked during this stretching exercise so that you don't encounter some type of injury.

Shoulder Flexions

Shoulder flexions are special stretching exercises where you are initially required to stay in a resting position, and from there, you must gently move your arms; first to your sides and then above your head, straight towards the ceiling.

Arm

Problems with your arms are inevitable these days, especially since most of the work you do is done while you are sitting and often with poor posture.

Arm Raise

- Keep your feet at a distance equal to that of your shoulders, and your arms should be resting at your sides. Maintain your palms with their face forward.
- Now, slowly start raising your arms to your sides until they reach about the height of your shoulders.
- Then, similarly, start lowering the arms slowly to the right, where you started.
- Maintain a constant breathing pattern throughout. You should also ensure that your hips are facing forward, and your spine is straight throughout.

Overhead Reach

- Maintain your feet at a distance that is slightly farther than shoulder-distance. However, the stance is not a big deal here because you can adjust it based on how you feel.
- Gently lift one arm up but make sure you don't bend back or forward. Keep the stretch position for a few seconds.
- Now, reach over to the other side. Repeat the same thing on each side four to five times.

Triceps Stretch

This stretching exercise can also be done both in sitting and standing positions.

- Maintain your stance at a hip-width distance and stand straight.
- Slowly lift one up to the top of your head towards the ceiling and then bend your elbow so that your right palm comes to the center portion of your back.
- Make sure the middle finger is resting along the length of the spinal cord.
- Now, take your other hand to gently grasp this elbow and push it downward.
- Hold this position for approximately 20 seconds and repeat the same on the other side.

Hand Stretch

Hand stretches are one of the best things to do if you feel like loosening up the muscles in your fingers after waking up in the morning.

- Stretch your hands in front of you and make sure your palms are facing in a downward direction.
- Open your palms and close them in a repeated motion and keep your fingers spread apart from each other.
- Repeat the same thing about 10 times, and while you are doing this, maintain normal breathing.

REPS AND REST IN STRENGTH TRAINING

This chapter has dealt with almost every important concept of strength training, but are you still unsure what to do after a workout is over? Well, you need to get enough rest to recover so that you can start the next day even fitter and stronger. Every workout stresses out the body in some way, which is why the number of reps you do and the amount of rest you take makes it even more important. This section will give you a better understanding of both these concepts.

Why Do You Need Rest After a Workout?

If you keep working out every day without taking a rest day in between, it can not only make you weak physically but also tire you out mentally. The main problem with not taking a rest day is that it decreases the amount of glycogen reserves in your muscles which, in turn, triggers your body to use up the proteins for energy (Fletcher, 2021). This means that your body no longer has sufficient protein for growth and repair.

Here's why rest is essential for seniors after workout sessions:

- On your rest days, the body works towards eliminating lactic acid from your body, which is the main culprit for muscle soreness.
- When you rest, your body also gets the chance to replenish the stores of glycogen, and when it doesn't get the chance to do this, you might feel fatigued.

- When you work out, your muscles will develop microscopic in them. It is on the rest days that your body will repair these tears.
- Excessive strain and repetitive stress on the same set of muscles increase the chance of injury.
- Exercising without rest also makes you mentally tired. When you feel exhausted, you are more likely to make poor decisions, which can lead to injuries. This is also another reason why rest days are important.

How Many Reps Are Appropriate For Seniors?

As I mentioned early in the book, strength training at least twice a week is a good place to start for seniors who are completely new to this. Now, as to how many reps you should be doing, anything in the range of 3 to 15 every set. When done in sets of 3, it can help you gain muscle mass, but make sure you take adequate rest between each of the sets. However, even if you do a single set in the beginning and then work your way up slowly, it can help you become stronger gradually. In fact, if you have health complications or joint problems, it is better that you start with a single set of 10 to 15 reps and practice that for a while before increasing the reps or sets or the amount of weight.

So now you have all the information to help start your journey to getting stronger. The next chapters will look into easy at-home strength training exercises for each muscle set. The next chapter focuses on the chest.

4

CHEST EXERCISES

> *The last three or four reps is what makes the muscle grow. This area of pain divides the champion from someone else who is not a champion. That's what most people lack, having the guts to go on and just say they'll go through the pain no matter what happens.*
>
> — ARNOLD SCHWARZENEGGER

This chapter suggests some basic chest strength training exercises for seniors that will help them become stronger and improve their overall health.

THE CHEST ANATOMY

Before you proceed to learn about the stretching exercises of the chest, it is important for you to know about the basic chest anatomy and the muscles that are present in this region, namely the serratus anterior, pectoralis minor, and pectoralis major.

The **pectoralis major** is one of the major muscles of the chest, and it takes the shape of a fan. The originating point of this muscle is near the sternum, ribs, and clavicle and travels all the way into the top portion of your humerus (Solari & Burns, 2020). This muscle is mostly used when you are engaging in forced inspiration. However, the opposite is not true; in the case of expiration, the muscle is not used. The main function of this muscle is that it helps in moving your arm towards your chest and, thus, in flexing the shoulder joint.

The **pectoralis minor** is a much thinner muscle and has a triangular shape, located just underneath the pectoralis major. The originating point of this muscle is between the third to fifth ribs of the ribcage, and it travels all the way up to the scapula. This muscle functions to stabilize the scapula (Baig & Bordoni, 2020).

Then we come to the **serratus anterior,** which is another muscle in the shape of a fan, but since its main part is deep under the pectoral muscles and scapula, it is often not considered a part of chest anatomy (Lung et al., 2022). It helps in the upward and forward movement of the scapula and keeps it stable.

The **intercostals** help form the chest wall and are present in between the ribs.

The **subclavius** is another set of small muscles that is triangular shaped and helps keep the first rib elevated. It is present across the shoulders.

LET'S BEGIN!

Some people think that chest exercises are all about that toned appearance, but it is more than that, especially for seniors. When your pectoral muscles are strong, it helps in maintaining good posture, gives support to the muscles and joints around it, and enhances the breathing procedure. But you must know which exercises you need to prioritize when you are starting out, so I have prepared a list for you.

Dumbbell Bench Press

This exercise works multiple joints at a time and is perfect for beginners.

Its benefits: Since this exercise is a unilateral movement, it is one of the best ones to improve imbalances in your muscle and correct your form. It also gives you much better contraction and a wider muscle stretch compared to a barbell. And it is not so stressful on the joints, making it perfect for seniors.

The muscles it targets: Anterior deltoids, pectoralis major, triceps, lateral deltoids, and rotator cuff.

Equipment required (if any): A set of dumbbells and a workout bench (an at-home alternative for the workout bench will do; this means you need a stable surface).

Warm-up: Try the stationary bike for about 10 to 15 minutes.

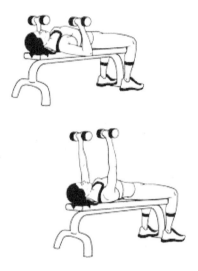

Steps to follow:

1. Lie on your back on the flat surface or the workout bench (whichever you are using) and hold a dumbbell of desired weight in each hand. Your arms need to be straight towards the ceiling on top of your chest. Keep your abs tightened and your feet planted firmly on the ground.
2. Now, gently lower the weights by bending your elbows and shoulders and bring them to the same level as your chest. If you cannot do that, bring them as low as you

comfortably can. Make sure you maintain a vertical posture in your forearms.
3. Push the weights back up and repeat.

Cool-down: You can either go for a slow walk or perform static stretches.

Safety tips: For starters, don't let the dumbbells collide when you lift them up; otherwise, it can cause your muscles to become insatiable. Don't start with very heavy weights right away. The dumbbells should not be hitting your chest too high; otherwise, you will be experiencing joint pain.

Reps and sets: Complete 3 sets of 10 reps each (in the beginning, you can do 2 sets).

Chest Flys

Its benefits: This exercise will help open the muscles of the chest and thus help deal with the tightness in your upper body, enhance your range of motion, and relieve upper back pain. It also strengthens your shoulder region and improves posture.

The muscles it targets: Triceps, shoulder, and chest.

Equipment required (if any): A set of dumbbells and a workout bench (an at-home alternative for the workout bench will do; this means you need a stable surface).

Warm-up: Perform arm swings. Keep your stance shoulder-width apart, your back straight, and then swing your arms.

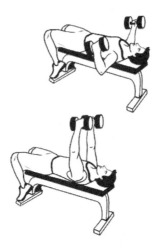

Steps to follow:

1. Lie down on the bench with a dumbbell in each hand. Your feet should be planted on the ground, and your back and head should remain on the bench throughout the course of the exercise.
2. Bend your elbows slightly and lift your arms above your head in a way that you don't lock them out. Your palms should be face-to-face with each other.
3. Take a deep breath and start lowering the dumbbells slowly but in an arc motion. Stop when you reach the level of your chest. Your arms should not be locked out completely, and they shouldn't go beyond your shoulders.
4. Breathe out and start bringing your arms back up again.

Cool-down: You can either go for a slow walk or perform side lunges.

Safety tips: Keep your shoulder blades on the floor and flat, even when you are bringing the dumbbells back up. While lowering the dumbbells, make sure you are not going beyond your shoulders. Both these situations have a chance of creating shoulder injury.

Reps and sets: Complete 3 sets of 10 to 15 reps each (in the beginning, you can do 2 sets).

Incline Pushups

Its benefits: The best thing about this exercise is that it helps you work on your chest muscles but, at the same time, doesn't put too much pressure on your elbows. It helps counteract a sagging spinal cord in seniors (Syed-Abdul et al., 2018).

The muscles it targets: Abs, chest, arms, and shoulders.

Equipment required (if any): A flat surface that is approximately 3 feet high.

Warm-up: Perform bent-arm wall stretch.

Steps to follow:

1. Maintain shoulder-distance between your hands and place them on an elevated flat surface. Form a straight line with your body, right from your shoulders to your heels.

2. Now, slowly bend your elbows so that you have a 45-degree angle with your main body. Start lowering your body until your elbows come at a parallel line with your back, and while doing this, inhale.
3. Return to the start position by extending your elbows. This will complete one rep.

Cool-down: You can either go for a slow walk or perform above-the-head stretches.

Safety tips: Don't place your hands too far from each other. Maintain a straight line with your body; otherwise, the effectiveness of this workout will be reduced. If you have a shoulder injury, you should talk to your healthcare provider before doing any type of pushups.

Reps and sets: Complete 3 sets of 10 reps each.

Chapter summary: Developing your chest muscles is all about *staying consistent* with your workout. If you are worried about equipment, then you can *start with pushups* since they not only develop the muscles of the chest but also engage your shoulders, upper back, and core. Just remember that you don't need to push yourself so hard that you feel uncomfortable with the weights because this increases your chances of injury. Also, *never skip warm-ups and cool-downs*. In the next chapter, we will be discussing strengthening your shoulder and arm muscles.

5

STRENGTHEN YOUR SHOULDERS AND ARMS

Did you know that you don't have to spend hours in the gym or pounding the pavement daily to maintain your fitness level? Simple shoulder and arm exercises in the comfort of your home are enough to keep your muscles strong, toned, and healthy.

THE SHOULDER AND ARM ANATOMY

There are about a set of 20 muscles present around your shoulder.

The four **rotator cuff muscles** in the shoulder are probably the most important ones since they allow you to rotate and turn your shoulder in multiple directions.

Then there are the **rhomboids,** whose main function is to assist you in lifting your shoulder blade. They start from the spine and end at the scapula.

The **trapezius** or **traps** muscle is present behind your shoulder and has a triangular shape. Its function is to help you lower and lift your shoulder.

Then there is the **deltoid** muscle that takes part in the backward, forward, and side movement of your arms and is present on the outside portion of your shoulder.

We will discuss the arm muscles in two parts: the forearm (between the elbow and the shoulder) and the upper arm (between the wrist and the elbow).

The *forearm muscles* are again of two types:

1. Superficial forearm muscles

    a. pronator teres
    b. flexor digitorum superficialis
    c. flexor carpi radialis
    d. palmaris longus
    e. flexor carpi ulnaris
    f. extensor carpi ulnaris
    g. extensor digiti minimi
    h. extensor digitorum communis
    i. extensor carpi radialis longus and brevis
    j. brachioradialis
    k. anconeus

2. Deep forearm muscles

   a. pronator quadratus
   b. flexor pollicis longus
   c. flexor digitorum profundus
   d. supinator
   e. extensor indicis
   f. extensor pollicis longus
   g. extensor pollicis brevis
   h. abductor pollicis longus

Next, we come to the **upper arm muscles**, which are mainly of four types:

1. triceps brachii
2. coracobrachialis
3. brachialis
4. biceps brachii

ARM EXERCISES

When you perform arm exercises, you slowly gain the power and strength necessary to perform your day-to-day activities all on your own, from lifting your groceries to engaging in hobbies like gardening.

Seated Bicep Curls With Dumbbells

Its benefits: It strengthens the forearms and the biceps.

The muscles it targets: Deltoids, forearms, and biceps.

Equipment required (if any): A set of dumbbells.

Warm-up: Try the arm raise.

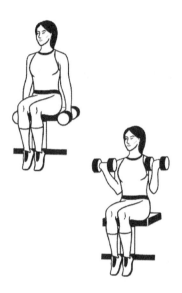

Steps to follow:

1. Sit on a chair with your back straight. It's best if the chair has a backrest. Take a dumbbell in each hand and allow your arms to hang along your sides, remaining close to your body.
2. Exhale and start bending your arms at the elbow while bringing the dumbbells all the way up to the top,

toward your chest. Your butt, shoulder, and head should remain in contact with the chair. After that, slowly lower your arms back to the initial position and inhale while doing so.

Cool-down: You can either perform arm raise or other static stretches.

Safety tips: The weight you lift must be comfortable and manageable for you; otherwise, you might encounter injury. Keep your shoulders stable.

Reps and sets: Complete 2 sets of 12 reps each.

Golfing

Its benefits: Older people often turn to casual walking as a form of physical activity, but research has proven that golfing might be even better in terms of the benefits (Kettinen et al., 2023). The research concluded that even though the exercise intensity of golf is not much, it tends to help people with a higher energy expenditure and continues for a longer duration, both of which have been seen to have a positive effect on glucose metabolism and lipid profile of elders. Apart from that, with golf, the elderly also get a chance of increased socialization, which is good for their mental health.

The muscles it targets: Back, chest, and forearms.

Equipment required (if any): Golf equipment.

Warm-up: Try the arm raise, shoulder rolls, and above-the-head stretch.

Cool-down: You can perform static stretches.

Safety tips: Always stretch before the game and remain hydrated throughout. Avoid playing out when the sun's rays are at its peak, and even while going out, don't forget your sunscreen.

Triceps Extension

Its benefits: It helps in building the muscles of your arms, increasing arm strength, and working the triceps (Maeo et al., 2022). When your triceps muscles are strong, it will automatically help you to have stronger elbow and shoulder joints (Landin et al., 2018). Did you know that your triceps are also important for activities as crucial as writing?

The muscles it targets: Pectoral, deltoids, and triceps.

Equipment required (if any): A set of dumbbells.

Warm-up: Try the triceps stretch.

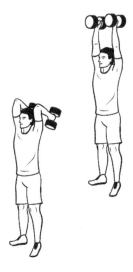

Steps to follow:

1. Your stance should be hip distance apart, and make sure you keep your left foot a little bit behind the right foot. Hold one dumbbell in each hand and cup them properly.
2. Slowly start lifting the dumbbells over your head. Engage your core and keep your shoulders relaxed.
3. Keep both your arms fully extended.
4. Exhale and start lowering the weights slowly. Bend your elbows and bring the dumbbells behind your head. Your back should not be arching at this point.
5. Once your elbows are at a 90-degree bend, inhale and start reversing the movement. When the dumbbell reaches the lowest position, it should not be touching the back of your head.

Cool-down: You can either do a triceps stretch, a light walk, or other static stretches.

Safety tips: Make sure you start with a weight that you are comfortable lifting in the initial stages because if you drop the dumbbells suddenly, it can cause injury. You should lift the dumbbells slowly and not try to speed up the process. Otherwise, it can cause tears in the muscles.

Reps and sets: Complete 2 sets of 12 reps each.

Gardening

Its benefits: Gardening not only has physical benefits but offers mental stimulation to the elderly too. It involves the usage of all motor skills and thus enhances flexibility and mobility in seniors.

The muscles it targets: Abdomen, back, neck, shoulders, arms, buttocks, and neck.

Equipment required (if any): Gardening equipment.

Safety tips: It's important that you use the right tools and keep your hands protected from direct contact with soil or fertilizer. Avoid going out in scorching heat, and make sure you do a little bit of warm-up before gardening so that you don't injure your muscles.

Swimming

Its benefits: Swimming is known to enhance cardiovascular health in the elderly and alleviates joint pain. It helps them work on all major muscles of the body and thus counteract muscle loss. Since swimming involves a lot of movements, it helps in enhancing flexibility. It also encourages socialization and thus benefits their mental health.

The muscles it targets: Lower back, core abdominal, shoulder, and forearm.

Warm-up: Perform arm circles in the pool.

Cool-down: You can perform some static hand stretches.

Safety tips: It's best that you walk carefully around the pool, reduce the chances of slippage. Avoid swimming alone; always have someone accompanying you. Know your swimming abilities. Do not try to cross your limit in order to show off. Before you dive, look out.

SHOULDER EXERCISES

Shoulder exercises play a major role in enhancing your independence. They can help you perform activities like lifting your grandkids up, reaching something that's on the top of the kitchen cupboard, or even something as basic as putting on your overcoat by yourself.

Shoulder Blade Squeezes

Its benefits: It helps in correcting your posture.

The muscles it targets: Rhomboids.

Warm-up: Try a light walk.

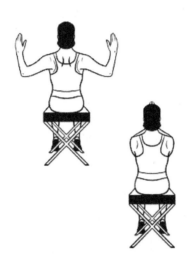

Steps to follow:

1. Place your arms by your sides and stand in a comfortable manner. Your spine position should be neutral.
2. Slowly bring your shoulders back. Start squeezing your shoulder blades and bring them close to each other.
3. Relax the shoulder blades and return to the neutral position.

Cool-down: Go for another light walk.

Safety tips: When bringing your shoulder blades together, make sure you are not arching your back. If, in the beginning, it seems difficult for you to do this exercise while standing, you can also consider doing it in the sitting position.

Reps and sets: Complete 3 sets of 10 reps each.

Arm Circles

Its benefits: It helps in toning the muscles in your arms and encourages more blood flow.

The muscles it targets: Biceps, triceps, and shoulders.

Warm-up: Try overhead reach.

Steps to follow:

1. Stand with your legs at a shoulder-width distance and then extend your arms parallel to the floor beneath.
2. Make constant, controlled motions in a circular fashion, with your arms in a forward direction. Try to make the circles bigger; you will feel the triceps muscles stretching a bit.
3. After continuing in this direction for about 10 seconds, reverse.

Cool-down: Triceps stretch.

Safety tips: Your breathing pattern should be deep and smooth, and your back should always be straight.

Reps and sets: Complete 3 sets of 15 to 20 reps each.

Wall Push-Ups

Its benefits: It enhances the upper body and corrects your posture; thus helps you perform better in your day-to-day activities with increased independence.

The muscles it targets: Shoulders, back, chest, and arms.

Warm-up: Try shoulder rolls.

Steps to follow:

1. Stand facing a wall with your feet shoulder-width apart and your arms extended, placing your palms on the wall at shoulder height.
2. Ensure that your hands are shoulder-width apart and your fingers are pointing upwards.
3. Keep your body straight, engage your core muscles, and maintain a comfortable distance from the wall.
4. Slowly bend your elbows and bring your chest towards the wall while inhaling.
5. Hold this position for 1–2 seconds, then exhale and push yourself back to the starting position.

Cool-down: Triceps stretch.

Safety tips: Your breathing pattern should be deep and smooth, and your back should always be straight.

Reps and sets: Complete 3 sets of 8 to 10 reps each.

Overhead Extension

Its benefits: It helps in improving body posture while putting little pressure on the wrists. It also helps in stabilizing your elbow and shoulder joints, which in turn helps you to lift heavy things. It also helps maintain the shape of the arms.

The muscles it targets: Triceps, core, and shoulders.

Equipment required (if any): Dumbbells.

Warm-up: Try triceps stretch.

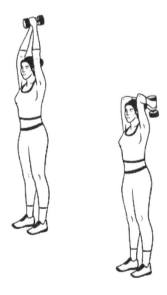

Steps to follow:

1. You can do this exercise either in a sitting or standing position. Use both your hands to hold the dumbbell above your head.

2. Now, start lowering the weight at the back of your head by bending your elbows very slowly. Try to lower the weight as much as you can, but your core must be engaged and your trunk upright. The weight should be brought down along the length of your spine.
3. When you have brought the weight to its lowest point, start bringing the weight back over your head by extending your elbows slowly.
4. Stay in this fully extended position for a few seconds, and then repeat the steps.

Cool-down: Shoulder rolls.

Safety tips: Ensure that you are not speeding up the exercise; otherwise, your muscles will get hurt. Use a weight that allows you to maintain good form but at the same time is a little bit challenging for you.

Reps and sets: Complete 3 sets of 15 reps each.

Chapter summary: Your arms and shoulder muscles are something that you will constantly be using throughout the day. So, whether it's about carrying around that heavy tote bag or fetching something from the top kitchen shelf, these muscles need to be strong. However, when you perform these exercises, *make sure you are not slumping forward*; otherwise, you will end up hurting your rotator cuff muscles. And finally, *never try to add a lot of weight too quickly to your workout routine*. In the next chapter, we will look at some basic leg, ankle, and foot strength training exercises for seniors that will help them become stronger and improve their overall health.

6

LEG, ANKLES, AND FEET EXERCISES

Don't let swollen and aching ankles prevent you from enjoying the physical activity your body needs and craves! There are many ways to modify legs, ankles, and feet exercises to make them safer and more comfortable. If your doctor approves it, take advantage of this opportunity to become more physically fit and enjoy the many benefits that come with it!

THE LEG ANATOMY

You have different muscles present in your lower and upper leg, and all these muscles together help you to flex your feet, stand on your toes, jump, run, and even walk. The muscles can be broadly divided into lower leg muscles, upper leg muscles, and foot muscles.

The upper leg muscles include:

- quadriceps
- hamstrings
- adductors

The lower leg muscles include:

- soleus
- gastrocnemius
- plantaris
- peroneus muscles
- tibialis muscles

The foot muscles include:

- flexors
- extensors
- tibialis peroneal
- tibialis anterior
- tibialis posterior

Well, I do understand that not everyone wants to run a marathon, but that's not why you need your lower body strength when you grow old. You also need it to walk short distances or perform everyday activities like getting up from the couch. Most people have this misconception that the lower body means quads, but there's so much more to it, as you probably might have understood from the leg anatomy we discussed above. So, here are some of the crucial benefits of building your lower body strength:

- When your leg muscles are strong, they will help you have better balance and keep you upright, thus reducing the risk of fall injuries.
- Your mobility will improve, and thus, you will be able to stay active, which will, in turn, provide you with a host of other benefits.
- The joints in your lower body undergo the maximum wear and tear however building strong muscles will keep them protected.

EXERCISES YOU SHOULD TRY

Your entire body is standing on the muscles present in your legs; thus, it is important that you focus on these large muscle groups that not only offer you balance but also dexterity.

Calf Raises

Its benefits: Calf raises are known to improve walking ability in seniors. Research shows that these exercises are also important for strengthening the ankles (Ema et al., 2017). Stronger calf muscles mean that doing basic day-to-day activities will no longer be a problem.

The muscles it targets: Gastrocnemius and soleus.

Equipment required (if any): Not applicable.

Warm-up: Walking.

Steps to follow:

1. Keep your feet at a distance equal to that of your shoulders and maintain a slight bend in your knees. Your abs should be pulled in and your back straight.
2. Start raising your heels but do it slowly and make sure your knees are extended. However, your knees should not be locked.
3. When you are standing on the tip of your toes, pause in that position for a second before coming back to the starting position.

Cool-down: Try foam rolling.

Safety tips: If you have recently encountered any type of lower-body injury, you should talk to your physical therapist before performing this exercise.

Reps and sets: Complete 3 sets of 15 reps each.

Knee Extensions

Its benefits: Knee extensions are known to reduce the risk of injury to your knee muscles and strengthen your thigh muscles. It also helps in enhancing your range of motion in the knees.

The muscles it targets: Quadriceps.

Equipment required (if any): Not applicable.

Warm-up: March in place for a minute.

Steps to follow:

1. Sit in a chair and keep your arms by your side and your feet flat on the surface below.
2. Straighten your right knee and extend it to its full length. This will put pressure on your quadriceps. Stay in this position for a few seconds.
3. Change legs and perform the same step.

Cool-down: Try foam rolling.

Safety tips: Don't jerk your leg while moving; otherwise, you will hurt your muscles.

Reps and sets: Complete the exercise 10 times on each leg.

Half Squats

Its benefits: Half squats enhance the range of motion and improve knee stability.

The muscles it targets: Hamstrings, quadriceps, calves, hip flexors, glutes, and core.

Equipment required (if any): A chair.

Warm-up: March in place for a minute.

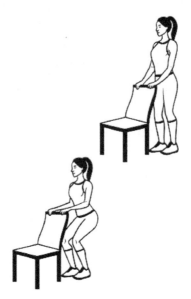

Steps to follow:

1. Keep your feet shoulder-distance apart and stand tall. Your toes should be facing slightly outwards.
2. To maintain balance, hold on to the chair and keep your arms outstretched in front of you.
3. Start sitting back as if you were sitting on a chair, and keep your core engaged while doing so. Don't go any lower than 45 degrees.
4. Your heels should be fixated on the surface throughout. Start standing back up and put equal pressure on both legs.

Cool-down: Try foam rolling.

Safety tips: Don't crane your neck while doing the squat because it can put unwanted pressure on your muscles. Keep your spine straight.

Reps and sets: Complete 2 sets of 10 reps each.

Chair Deadlift

Its benefits: It immensely helps in strengthening your hamstrings and glutes.

The muscles it targets: Calves, hips, quads, glutes, back, and core.

Equipment required (if any): A chair and resistance bands.

Warm-up: A light jog.

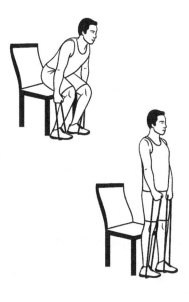

Steps to follow:

1. Place the resistance bands on the floor and then sit on the chair with a straight posture.
2. Your feet should be shoulder-distance apart on the resistance band. Maintain the toes at an angle pointed slightly outwards.
3. Reach down and hold the resistance band but maintain a straight posture while doing so, with your chest up and shoulders back and down. Your arms should also be straight while holding on to the resistance band.
4. Now, while you are holding on to the resistance band, stand up. When you come to the top position of the movement, ensure that you squeeze your buttocks and keep your knees and hips straight.
5. Sit back down slowly and repeat.

Cool-down: Try foam rolling.

Safety tips: Ensure that you don't move your knees during the exercise, and you are keeping equal weight in both legs.

Reps and sets: Complete 2 sets of 10 reps each.

Ankle Circles

Its benefits: It helps release the tension and stress that accumulates in your ankles, and it opens the ankle joints.

The muscles it targets: Calves.

Equipment required (if any): Not applicable.

Warm-up: A light jog.

Steps to follow:

1. Stand straight and keep your arms by your sides. Your feet should be kept at hip distance apart.
2. Slowly shift the weight of your body on your right leg and then start pointing the toes of your left foot to the ground.
3. Rotate your left foot slowly and make small circles with the help of your ankle.
4. Repeat the same step by alternating the legs.

Cool-down: March in place.

Safety tips: In the beginning, perform smaller circles and then make wider ones to open your ankle joints. In case you feel any kind of discomfort, make sure you revert to smaller circles.

Reps and sets: Complete 3 sets of 30 seconds on each foot.

Step Up

Its benefits: One of the most crucial benefits of performing this exercise is that it enhances leg strength and improves stability.

The muscles it targets: Hamstrings, quadriceps, and buttocks.

Equipment required (if any): A bench or a sturdy elevated surface.

Warm-up: A light jog in place.

Steps to follow:

1. Stand in front of the elevated surface that you have chosen to work with. Raise your right foot and place it on the surface.
2. Step up onto the surface (stair or bench) by putting your entire weight onto your right foot. Simultaneously, bring your left foot up so that both your feet are on the elevated surface.
3. Step down with your right foot and then your left, to return to the starting position.
4. Perform 10 steps while leading with the left foot and 10 steps while leading with the right. This completes one set.

Cool-down: March on the spot.

Safety tips: Make sure that the elevated surface on which you are stepping is sturdy and does not have the chance to cause any fall injuries.

Reps and sets: Complete 3 sets.

Hip Extensions

Its benefits: This exercise supports your lower back while enhancing the stability and strength of your glutes.

The muscles it targets: Gluteus and hamstrings.

Equipment required (if any): A chair.

Warm-up: A light jog in place.

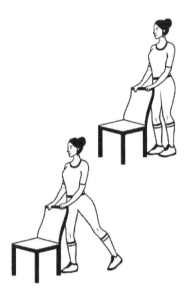

Steps to follow:

Stand in front of a chair (with the back of the chair facing you) with your back straight and shoulders wide apart. Your knees should be locked in position and straight.

1. Now, hold the chair with both hands for stability during the exercise.
2. Without arching your back, try to extend your right hip towards the back.
3. Slowly return your foot to the original position and repeat the same movement 10 times.
4. Then, change legs and repeat 10 times.

Cool-down: Try foam rolling.

Safety tips: Maintain good form so that you don't hurt yourself.

Reps and sets: Complete 3 sets.

Side Leg Raise

Its benefits: This exercise mainly helps in building the strength of the outer thighs and hip abductor muscles.

The muscles it targets: Gluteus, hamstrings, lower back, hip flexors, and core.

Equipment required (if any): A chair.

Warm-up: A light jog.

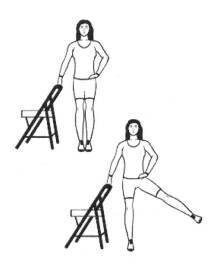

Steps to follow:

Keep your feet slightly apart, maintain a straight spine, and stand behind a chair.

1. Use the support of the chair while you slowly lift your right leg to the sides. Your toes should be facing forward during this movement, and your back must be straight.
2. Then, slowly return your right leg to the initial position and repeat the same movement with the left leg.

Cool-down: March on the spot.

Safety tips: Maintain good form so that you don't hurt yourself.

Reps and sets: Complete 2 sets of 10 reps for each leg.

Chapter summary: If you want to *maintain an active lifestyle even after retirement,* working on your lower body strength is extremely important. This will make performing everyday activities like bending or squatting, walking up and down the stairs, and standing for a long time much easier. It will also *reduce the chances of experiencing fall injuries and decrease stiffness and pain in the muscles.* In the next chapter, I will suggest some basic upper and lower back strength training exercises for seniors that are especially important for people who have spent a major portion of their life performing a desk job.

7

LET'S STRENGTHEN THE BACK

The human body is like a river, with the force of gravity pulling us ever downward. We can often feel the strain that comes from being subject to this relentless force, as it brings weariness and pain to our muscles, joints, and bones. But with the gentle power of back stretches and strength training exercises, we can reverse this flow, easing pain and tension as we move towards a greater sense of well-being.

THE BACK ANATOMY

There are approximately 40 muscles present in your back (Holloway, 2021). I have divided the muscles into different categories based on their functionality so that it is easier for you to understand.

First, let's have a look at the *muscles that mainly help move the head*.

- sternocleidomastoid
- splenius capitis
- semispinalis capitis
- longissimus capitis

Then, there are the *muscles that help move the shoulders.*

- rhomboids
- trapezius
- levator scapulae

After that, let's see the names of the *muscles that are responsible for the movement of the upper arms.*

- supraspinatus
- infraspinatus
- latissimus dorsi
- teres minor
- teres major

Next, there are *muscles that assist in the movement of the spine.*

- quadratus lumborum
- sacrospinalis

Last but not least, there are *muscles that help in moving the upper legs.*

- psoas minor
- iliopsoas

Now that you have a better idea about the back anatomy, it's crucial that you understand why you need to train your back muscles as you age. If you have had a sedentary lifestyle for most of your life, for example, a job that required you to sit all day, then your muscles must have become stiff and gained fat by now. In fact, a study has also reported that 75% out of the 64 call center employees that were examined suffered from back pain (Bontrup et al., 2019). But when you perform back strengthening exercises, they give you relief from the pain, improve posture, and give you better flexibility.

LOWER BACK EXERCISES

Try these lower back exercises for a few days, and you will notice the difference yourself.

Curl Ups

Its benefits: This exercise helps in enhancing back support, gives you stability, strengthens your core, relieves you of back pain, and improves your posture.

The muscles it targets: Neck, chest, hip flexors, obliques, and core.

Equipment required (if any): Yoga mat.

Warm-up: Overhead reach.

Steps to follow:

1. Lie down on a yoga mat with your feet flat on the ground and knees bent. Your feet must be kept slightly away from your buttocks.
2. In order to fix your neck position, slowly bring your chin closer to your chest and curl your head.
3. Place your hands behind your ears, and your elbows should be pointing outwards to the sides.
4. Slowly bring your upper back off the floor at 30 to 40 degrees. At this point, your neck, legs, arms, and shoulders should be relaxed because it's your abs that are pulling you up.
5. Pause for a second and lower your body back to its original position.

Cool-down: Above-the-head stretch.

Safety tips: You shouldn't be doing this exercise within one hour of waking up; otherwise, you will have a high chance of injuring your muscles. For better motor control and a lesser risk of injury, perform this exercise at a speed you are comfortable with and progressively increase.

Reps and sets: Complete 2 sets of 10 reps.

Cat and Camel

Its benefits: This exercise strengthens the core and back muscles, reduces stiffness, increases flexibility, and fixes poor posture.

The muscles it targets: Back, shoulders, arms, and neck.

Equipment required (if any): Yoga mat.

Warm-up: Bent-arm wall stretch.

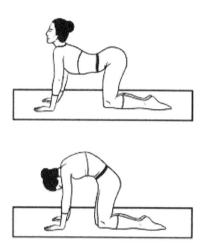

Steps to follow:

Place your hands and knees on the yoga mat; at this point, your spine should be in a neutral position.

1. Slowly bring your head down and round your back up. It's very similar to a cat arching its back.
2. Now, reverse the movement by relaxing your back and imitating the valley between the humps of a camel.
3. Once both movements are done, return to your initial position and repeat.

Cool-down: Shoulder rolls.

Safety tips: Perform this exercise only when you are sure that you will be able to get back up from the floor. If you feel pain in your wrists while doing this exercise, consider lowering yourself down to your elbows.

Reps and sets: Complete 2 sets of 10 reps.

Pelvic Tilts

Its benefits: This exercise will help you build strong buttocks and abdominal muscles. It is also a great stretching exercise for the back and reduces stiffness in the lower back. If you are suffering from lower back pain, this is one of the best exercises to perform.

The muscles it targets: Lower back and abdominal muscles.

Equipment required (if any): Yoga mat.

Warm-up: March on the spot.

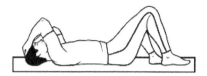

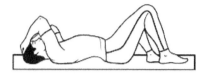

Steps to follow:

1. Lie down on the yoga mat and bend your knees while keeping your feet flat on the surface.
2. Now that you are in a neutral position, you can slowly lift your lower back off the yoga mat simply with the help of the natural curve that's present in your lumbar region.
3. Gently rock your hips in the direction of your head while you exhale.
4. Stay in this position for a few seconds. Then, inhale and return to your starting position.

Cool-down: Extended child's pose.

Safety tips: Breathing is integral for your body to realize the full benefits of this exercise. Engage your core muscles properly, but don't try to pressure yourself into doing anything.

Reps and sets: Complete 2 sets of 10 reps.

Sit-Back

Its benefits: This exercise helps stabilize the lower back region in the elderly. As you do this exercise and gain better control over your core muscles, it will help in improving balance and postural stability.

The muscles it targets: Lower back and abdominal muscles.

Equipment required (if any): Yoga mat.

Warm-up: Side lying parallel arm chest stretch.

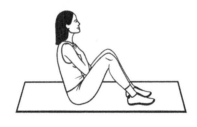

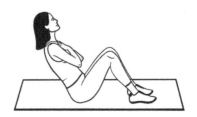

Steps to follow:

Sit on the yoga mat with your arms folded over your chest and knees bent.

1. Start slowly sitting back to a distance that you comfortably can. During this movement, make sure you are not over-stressing your back muscles.
2. Then, return to your initial position and repeat.

Cool-down: Extended child's pose.

Safety tips: If your feet are coming off the floor while performing the exercise, you need to stop. As you sit back, you need to maintain a straight spine.

Reps and sets: Complete 2 sets of 10 reps.

Hip Flexion

Its benefits: This exercise enhances the range of motion at the hips while helping you to maintain good posture. It also assists in building strong hip flexor muscles. Whether you are reaching the top of a cupboard, trying to carry your own bag on your next trip, or doing the laundry, this exercise will make these daily activities a breeze.

The muscles it targets: Abs and hips.

Equipment required (if any): Yoga mat.

Warm-up: Shoulder press-ups.

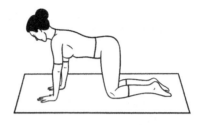

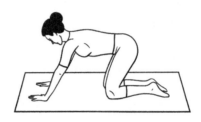

Steps to follow:

1. Position your body on your knees and hands on the yoga mat. Your hips and back must be in a neutral position.
2. Keep your back as straight as you can while slowly moving your hips backward.
3. Then, return to the initial position and repeat.

Cool-down: Extended child's pose.

Safety tips: Maintain steady breathing throughout the exercise. Don't push your hips too much if it hurts your muscles.

Reps and sets: Complete 2 sets of 10 reps.

UPPER BACK EXERCISES

Now that you have learned a few lower back exercises, let's look at how you can train your upper back.

Banded Pull-Aparts

Its benefits: This exercise keeps your shoulders in good health, enhances upper body strength, and improves mobility.

The muscles it targets: Rhomboids, rotator cuffs, and trapezius.

Equipment required (if any): Resistance band.

Warm-up: Arm raise.

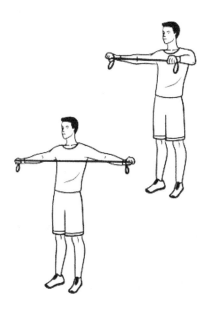

Steps to follow:

1. Stand straight, keep your feet shoulder-distance apart, and maintain a slight bend in your knees.
2. Hold a shoulder-width resistance band and bring your arms slowly in front of you. Your palms should be facing downwards while doing this.
3. Pull the band apart with both your arms. Pull as far as your muscles allow you to hold in the extended position for a second, and then return back to your initial position.

Cool-down: Above-the-head stretch.

Safety tips: Maintain a stable breathing pattern as you do this exercise. If your muscles feel overly achy, you should consider taking a step back to rest.

Reps and sets: Complete 3 sets of 10 reps.

Seated Row

Its benefits: This exercise helps strengthen the back and upper arm muscles. It also helps the elderly regain their balance and build back their posture.

The muscles it targets: Upper back muscles and latissimus dorsi.

Equipment required (if any): A chair.

Warm-up: Arm raises

Steps to follow:

1. Sit on the chair while maintaining a straight posture.
2. Extend your arms to their full length in front of you.
3. Now, squeeze your shoulder blades together while pulling your elbows back.
4. Throughout this exercise, your chest should be up. Return your arms to their initial position and repeat.

Cool-down: Above-the-head stretch.

Safety tips: Sit straight; otherwise, you will only be promoting poor spinal positioning throughout the exercise.

Reps and sets: Complete 3 sets of 10 reps.

Bent-Over Dumbbell Rear Delt Row

Its benefits: It's a great exercise to build stability in your shoulders and strengthen the muscles of your back. It can also protect you from strain if you know how to brace your abs and position your back during this exercise.

The muscles it targets: Upper and lower back muscles.

Equipment required (if any): Dumbbells.

Warm-up: Arm raise.

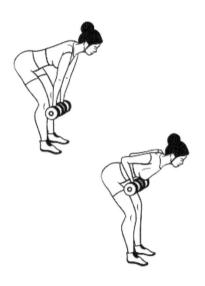

Steps to follow:

1. Stand straight and keep a slight bend in your knees, with your legs shoulder-distance apart.
2. Pick up a dumbbell in each hand and make sure both your palms are facing each other.
3. Slowly bend over, approximately at a 45-degree angle, and inhale.
4. Start pulling the dumbbells up until they reach the side of your chest, and while doing this, exhale. Lift the dumbbells only to the point your range of motion comfortably allows you to.
5. Once you have reached the top position, start lowering the weights back to the starting position in a controlled manner. Inhale during the process.
6. Stay bent until you complete all your reps.

Cool-down: Above-the-head stretch.

Safety tips: Don't move your wrists too much during this exercise, or else you might hurt yourself. It is a sign that you are lifting too much weight if you have a hard time maintaining good posture during the exercise.

Reps and sets: Complete 2 sets of 10 reps.

Chapter summary: Standing up or sitting down are day-to-day movements that many seniors struggle with over time. If you are one of them, you need to work on your lower back. There might be days when you might feel that getting out of bed is the most challenging task you ever had to do because of the excruciating back pain, but all of this can be things of the past with some simple back exercises that have been discussed in this chapter. *Back exercises can significantly reduce back pain, reduce the risk of injuries, and enhance your quality of life.* In the next chapter, I will discuss some basic core strength training exercises for seniors.

8

BUILD YOUR STRENGTH, FROM THE CORE

> *If it doesn't challenge you, it doesn't change you.*
>
> — FRED DEVITO

If you thought that core-building exercises were only meant for athletes and people under the age of 30, it's time for you to rethink because as you age, it's your core muscles that you will need to do some of the most basic activities in your everyday life. In general, if your core is not strong, you will face issues related to mobility and balance, both of which can increase your tendency to incur fall injuries. So, if you are ready to build a stronger core, let's get started.

THE CORE ANATOMY

Before we get into the different exercises, it's important that you have a brief idea about the muscles of the core.

These muscles can be divided into two parts: the core hip muscles, and the core trunk muscles.

The core hip muscles further include the following:

- abductors
- extensors
- adductors
- hip flexors
- rotators

The core trunk muscles on the other hand, comprise of these:

- abdominals
- lumbar
- thoracolumbar
- lateral thoracolumbar

Now, let's talk about why seniors need to work on their core muscles. According to a study published in the *Journal of Orthopaedic & Sports Physical Therapy,* there is a correlation between increased age and poor quality of core back muscles, which is why intervention in the form of strength training is essential (Sions et al., 2017). Core exercises will help you stay upright and improve your flexibility. These exercises are also great for people who have been struggling with arthritis.

Everyday movements like turning, lifting, and bending will become much easier after you incorporate core strengthening exercises into your routine.

EXERCISES YOU SHOULD TRY

According to a review of studies published in 2015, over 50% of the people in the U.S. suffer from issues related to back pain (Chang et al., 2015). If you don't want to fall in that bracket, here are some exercises you should try at home.

The Superman

Its benefits: The superman exercise is known to reduce the risk of injuries, helps in building good posture, and supports the spine.

The muscles it targets: Abdominal muscles, lower back, hamstrings, glutes, and shoulders.

Equipment required (if any): Yoga mat.

Warm-up: Bent-arm wall stretch.

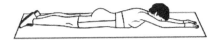

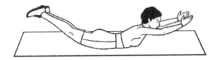

Steps to follow:

1. Lie down on the yoga mat while keeping your face down. Keep your legs straight and extend your arms in front of you. Your head should be in a neutral position; that is, you should not try to look up.
2. Slowly lift your legs and arms off the yoga mat to about six inches off the surface or until your lower back permits. Stay in this position for a couple of seconds. It should look like a flying Superman.
3. After that, bring your arms and legs back to the surface slowly and repeat.

Cool-down: Above-the-head stretch.

Safety tips: Keep in mind that you should be lifting your body to a height that you feel comfortable with and not farther than that. Avoid looking up or extending your neck too much because this can lead to pain and discomfort.

Reps and sets: Complete 3 sets of 10 reps.

The Bridge

Its benefits: The bridge targets muscles of the body that will enhance your strength and power and ease pain in the lower back region.

The muscles it targets: Hamstrings, abdominal muscles, and glutes.

Equipment required (if any): Yoga mat.

Warm-up: Above-the-head stretch.

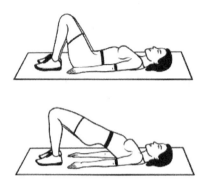

Steps to follow:

1. Lie down on a yoga mat with your hands resting on your sides. Bend your knees and keep your feet flat on the surface.
2. Tighten your buttock and abdominal muscles; for this, you can push your lower back into the yoga mat.
3. Slowly start raising your hips to the point where you form a straight line from your shoulder to your knees.
4. Pull your belly button back by squeezing your core muscles.
5. Stay in this position for about 10 seconds.
6. Start lowering the hips slowly to return to the initial position.

Cool-down: Arm raise.

Safety tips: Don't extend your lower back too much, as this will raise your hips too high and cause strain on the muscles.

Reps and sets: Complete 3 sets of 10 seconds each.

Reverse Lowers

Its benefits: If you want to make lifting something easier, then this is the exercise that you need to perform.

The muscles it targets: Hamstrings, abdominal muscles, and lower back.

Equipment required (if any): Mat or Yoga mat, Folded towel

Warm-up: Shoulder rolls.

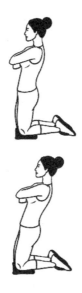

Steps to follow:

1. Kneel on the floor (use a folded towel under knees for comfort). Your feet should be on the floor and knees shoulder-distance apart. Keep your arms crossed on your chest.
2. Slowly lean back, lowering down but keep your trunk stiff. Don't push yourself too much. You should lower yourself only as much as your range of motion allows you to. When you reach the end position, pause for a few seconds.
3. Then, raise your body back to the initial position and repeat.

Cool-down: Arm raise.

Safety tips: Perform fewer reps if it feels too stressful on the muscles, or you can shorten the distance that you are leaning back.

Reps and sets: Complete 3 sets of 10 reps.

Bird Dog

Its benefits: Bird dog is an excellent exercise to give you relief from lower back pain, encourage your body to maintain a neutral spine, improve your range of motion, and enhance stability.

The muscles it targets: Quads, abs, glutes, and lower back.

Equipment required (if any): Yoga mat.

Warm-up: Arm raise.

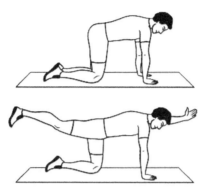

Steps to follow:

1. Kneel down on the yoga mat and keep your knees at a hip distance apart from one another. Bring your hands down on the yoga mat too and keep them shoulder-distance apart.
2. Slowly lift one arm and extend it in front of you. Lift the opposite leg behind you. The leg and the arm should form a straight line.
3. Stay in this position for a few seconds and then return to the starting position on your hands and knees. Switch arms and legs and repeat—complete five reps for each side, which will make one set.

Cool-down: March on the spot.

Safety tips: If you are not able to maintain good form when you are starting out, instead of lifting the arm and leg together, do them one by one. When you feel that you are steady enough, you can do them together.

Reps and sets: Complete 3 sets of 10 reps.

Side Bends

Its benefits: The side bends are an extremely easy exercise that you can perform to strengthen your abs, enhance breathing, and promote better posture.

The muscles it targets: Oblique Abs.

Equipment required (if any): Chair.

Warm-up: Arm raise.

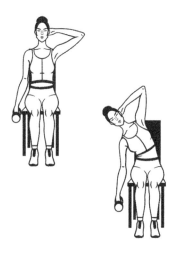

Steps to follow:

1. Sit on a chair with your feet planted firmly on the surface below and keep them at hip-width apart.
2. You should lean a little bit forward so that you don't tend to hunch during the exercise.
3. Slowly raise your right arm over your head and simultaneously bend your upper body to the left side as if you are trying to reach something. While you are bending, your upper body should not twist to the sides and must always be facing forward.
4. Remain in this stretched position for about 20 seconds and then return to the initial position. Repeat by switching sides.

Cool-down: Shoulder rolls.

Safety tips: Don't hunch your shoulders; otherwise, you will hurt your back muscles.

Reps and sets: Complete 3 sets of 6 reps (3 on each side).

Heel Slides

Its benefits: Heel slides are known to help you build trunk stability and lower body mobility. It also tones the leg and abdominal muscles when performed correctly with good posture and improves the flow of blood in these regions.

The muscles it targets: Abs, knees, and hips.

Equipment required (if any): Yoga mat.

Warm-up: A light jog.

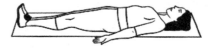

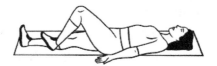

Steps to follow:

1. Lie down on the yoga mat and keep your feet on the surface with your knees bent. Try to draw your belly button inside by tightening your abdominal muscles.
2. Slide your left heel slowly toward your buttocks and bend the knee. Your aim should be to use your heel to touch the buttocks, but if you aren't able to, that's okay —you need not push yourself too hard.
3. When you have bent your knee to the maximum point, hold for 5 seconds before returning to the starting position, and then repeat with the other leg.

Cool-down: Go for a walk.

Safety tips: Don't overexert your leg muscles by trying to pull them back too much.

Reps and sets: Complete 3 sets of 10 reps (5 on each side).

Chapter summary: *Core strength is something you need in all stages of your life.* When you are performing these exercises for about two weeks, you will start noticing changes in your muscles. But in order to avoid bad posture and injury, *you should keep in mind not to perform any sudden jerky movements.* Moreover, if you are using a chair for your exercise, it should be sturdy. When you work on your core, the other muscles of your body learn to function in harmony. In the next chapter, I will discuss some basic abdominal strength training exercises for seniors that are specifically directed toward training your abs and not the other muscles in your core region.

9

THE ABDOMINALS

> *A fit, healthy body—that is the best fashion statement.*
>
> — JESS C. SCOTT

The core involves a lot of muscles right from the rib cage down to your hips, but in this chapter, we are only going to focus on the abdominal muscles and what you can do to train them.

THE ABDOMINAL ANATOMY

Like we did in all other chapters before this, we will first look at the abdominal anatomy before discussing any exercise so that you know what muscles you are dealing with. There are five major muscles in this region. Of these five, three are flat muscles, whereas two are vertical muscles (Cleveland Clinic, n.d.).

The flat muscles are as follows:

- **External obliques:** These are a pair of muscles that run along the side of the abdomen. When you twist your body from one side to another, it is because of these muscles.
- **Internal obliques:** They are present just on top of the external obliques and also help in twisting your body from side to side.
- **Transversus abdominis:** Right at the bottom of the stack of flat muscles are the transversus abdominis. Their function is to help maintain the right internal abdominal pressure and stabilize the body.

The vertical muscles are as follows:

- **Rectus abdominis:** This muscle starts right from the center of the abdomen and travels down to the pelvis. It functions to keep your internal organs in place. The bumps on the abdomen that you see in someone having a "six-pack" is because of the rectus abdominis.
- **Pyramidalis:** This triangle-shaped muscle is comparatively smaller, and its exact location is very low in your pelvic region. It's associated with maintaining the right level of internal pressure in your abdomen.

EXERCISES YOU SHOULD TRY

Now that we have learned about the basic anatomy of the abdominal region, let's look at some of the exercises that you can perform on a daily basis to strengthen these muscles.

Dead Bug

Its benefits: As funny as the name of this exercise may seem, it's one of the best ones you can do for your abs, especially when you want to train the deeper muscles present within. It doesn't take much to lose control of your core as you age, but this exercise will improve your stability and control.

The muscles it targets: Spinal erectors and transverse abdominis.

Equipment required (if any): Yoga mat.

Warm-up: A light jog.

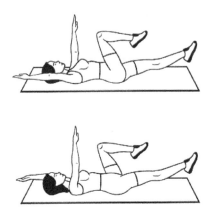

Steps to follow:

1. Lie down on the yoga mat and raise your arms over your chest so that there is a 90-degree angle between your torso and the arms. Lift your feet from the ground and bend your hips and knees, too, so that you have another 90-degree angle here. This will be your initial position for the exercise.
2. Your left leg and right arm should remain in the position that they are currently in. Slowly start reaching backward with your left arm towards the floor, and at the same time, extend your right hip and knee. Stop just before either your leg or the arm touches the ground. At that moment, reverse and return to your initial position.
3. Now, perform the same steps on your opposite leg and arm.

Cool-down: Arm raise.

Safety tips: Don't overexert your muscles, and don't move too fast during this exercise, especially when you are a beginner.

Reps and sets: Complete 3 sets of 10 reps (5 on each side).

Modified Plank

Its benefits: One of the main benefits of performing a modified plank is that it helps in reducing lower back pain. It also builds good posture, which, in turn, alleviates the chances of developing back pain in the future.

The muscles it targets: Abs, shoulder, arm, and core.

Equipment required (if any): Yoga mat.

Warm-up: A light jog.

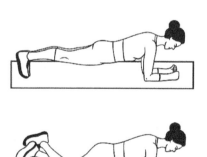

Steps to follow:

1. Lie down on the yoga mat with your stomach facing downwards. Raise yourself up slowly so that your body is resting on your knees and forearms.
2. Keep your neck and head aligned with your back, and your elbows and shoulders should be in a straight line. Engage your abdominal muscles.
3. Press your knees and elbows towards one another, which will create resistance. However, none of the body parts should move from their positions. Hold this position for about 10 seconds.
4. Return to the initial position and repeat.

Cool-down: Shoulder flexions.

Safety tips: Don't let your spinal cord sag during this exercise.

Reps and sets: Complete 3 sets.

Seated Knee Lifts

Its benefits: This exercise keeps the knee muscles flexible and thus helps seniors in dealing with reduced mobility issues at this age that takes away their independence.

The muscles it targets: Abs, glutes, and hip flexors.

Equipment required (if any): Chair.

Warm-up: A light jog.

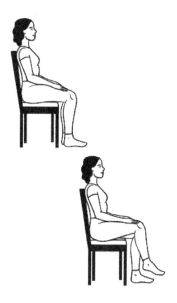

Steps to follow:

1. Sit comfortably on a chair with your feet planted firmly on the ground at hip distance apart and your spine straight.
2. If it feels more comfortable for you, you can grip the chair seat just below your thighs.
3. Slowly start lifting one knee and gradually bring it toward your chest as much as you can. If you have lifted your foot about 6 inches from the ground, then stop.
4. Start lowering the foot back onto the ground and repeat with the other leg.

Cool-down: March on the spot.

Safety tips: Don't keep raising your knee if it is putting too much pressure on your muscles and you feel too much pain.

Reps and sets: Complete 3 sets of 10 reps (5 on each leg).

Reverse Crunch

Its benefits: If you want good posture, stability, balance, reduced back pain, and strong ab muscles, then this exercise is exactly what you should try.

The muscles it targets: Abs.

Equipment required (if any): Yoga mat.

Warm-up: Extended child's pose.

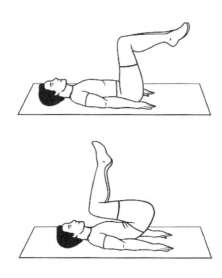

Steps to follow:

1. Lie down on your back on the yoga mat and keep your arms along your sides.
2. Now, bend your knee and bring your legs up so that your hips and knees are along the same line and the lower legs are parallel to the surface. Your spine should remain stuck to the ground firmly and maintain a neutral position.
3. Curl your knees and hips toward your chest and exhale as you perform this contraction. Hold this position for a second and then slowly return to the initial position while inhaling.

Cool-down: March on the spot.

Safety tips: Your shoulders and neck should remain on the mat in a relaxed manner. When you are drawing your knees towards your chest, avoid doing so with the help of momentum and instead do it with your ab muscles.

Reps and sets: Complete 3 sets of 10 reps.

Seated Forward Roll-Ups

Its benefits: It enhances strength, flexibility, and stability and helps in improving coordination.

The muscles it targets: Abs.

Equipment required (if any): Chair.

Warm-up: Arm raise.

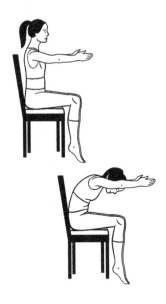

Steps to follow:

1. Sit on the chair and extend your feet in front of you. Your heels should be touching the floor.
2. Keep your arms straight out in front of you, angled properly with your legs. Maintain as much upright posture as you can.
3. Inhale and bring your chin towards your chest. Your legs should be straight at this point.
4. Exhale while you bend your entire torso towards your toes.
5. Go the furthest you can and when you can't anymore, breathe in and return to the initial position.
6. Repeat.

Cool-down: Shoulder rolls.

Safety tips: Keep in mind that if you want to reap the benefits of this exercise, then you must move slowly. It's not momentum that should be pushing your body forward, but your abs that should be doing the work.

Reps and sets: Complete 3 sets of 10 reps.

Chapter summary: What comes to your mind when you picture someone working on their abs? Probably someone doing a lot of crunches, right? Well, that doesn't have to be the case because building abs are not only about appearance, as most people make it look like nowadays. *It is also about performing day-to-day activities with ease.* And remember, just because you want to work on your abdomen doesn't mean you will hammer in a lot of planks and sit-ups into your routine. You need to be mindful of your age and your goals and devise a plan accordingly.

CONCLUSION

> *The longer I live, the more beautiful life becomes. If you foolishly ignore beauty, you will soon find yourself without it. Your life will be impoverished. But if you invest in beauty, it will remain with you all the days of your life.*
>
> — FRANK LLOYD WRIGHT

If you ask any aged person their views on muscle strength, they will all probably tell you the same thing: it will fade with age and is not stagnant. But it definitely doesn't mean that you will sit and do nothing about it.

Research has proven the relationship between a decrease in muscle mass and age (Landers et al., 2001). However, at the same time, research has also shown that strength training can help seniors combat muscle loss and become stronger (Seguin

& Nelson, 2003). In fact, this can make performing everyday tasks so much easier that you no longer have to depend on others for the most mundane activities.

If you have reached this conclusion, then you have already read about the benefits and several strength training exercises that you can try at home. But one thing that I want to remind you once again is that when you are starting out, it can be very tempting indeed to feel like lifting heavier weights, but that's where you need to practice a little bit of restraint. When you get too excited and lift heavier weights than you can handle, you are putting yourself on the path of injury. So, how can you make your training sessions fun yet safe? When one type of movement gets too easy for you, try to increase the rep ranges. Keep in mind that building strength is the goal, but increasing the weight is not always the way to get there; sometimes, there are alternatives too.

Next, always remember that performing the exercises with correct form and posture is essential. So, when you are practicing some new form of exercise, it is advisable that you do so by looking at yourself in the mirror so that you understand where the form is going wrong.

But if you have not been exercising because you thought your body was too weak for this or if you had been advised by a random person not to exercise because of an injury you had incurred a long time back, it's highly likely that this is your fear talking. Regular exercise will only do good to your body, and in fact, if you were someone who mostly led a sedentary lifestyle until now, then strength training is an absolute must for your routine.

If you have been looking forward to growing old with grace and vitality, then all you need to do is follow the steps mentioned in this book, and within a few weeks, you will learn the secret of active aging. Your abdominal muscles or your back muscles might be compromised or weak right now because of some surgery or injury, but that's completely fine. This book has discussed exercises for people in all stages of their lives.

This book will not only teach you how to perform these exercises in a step-by-step manner, but each chapter also breaks down the muscles of those portions of the body. In addition to that, there are also several stretching exercises that you can perform for warm-ups and cool-downs. As you keep strengthening your muscles, you can come back to this book whenever you want so that you can learn to strengthen the rest.

Every exercise that has been described in this book comes with its own set of descriptions in the form of benefits, how to perform the exercise, the equipment you need, safety tips, the number of sets, and so on. You can use this book in any way you want. You can either pick exercises from each chapter to decide your own workout routine or even work through every chapter systematically. All you need to finish this book is a little bit of effort and patience, and in the end, a strong body and more independence await you!

Aging is inevitable. You cannot stop this process. But you don't necessarily have to lose strength and muscle mass just because you have reached a certain age. If you take a step towards educating yourself about how your body works and the actions you can take to prevent muscle loss, then you are already one step ahead of the others in terms of working towards a better you. So, pick a few at-home exercises from within these pages and start your journey to aging strongly, one step at a time. Still feeling that the exercises are too tough? Why not simply start with the stretching exercises and then work your way to the bodyweight exercises and slowly move towards the weight training exercises involving resistance bands and dumbbells? I'm sure it won't be too overwhelming for you that way.

If you have been suffering from some chronic illness, it's better that you consult your physician before embarking on any exercise routine. But if you get the go-ahead from them, start your strength training today. Don't worry about injuries because you can keep them at bay with proper technique and some simple safety tips that I have already included in the book. And what's more is that when you exercise regularly, it reduces your chances of falling by 23% (Manor, 2019)!

If this book has answered your queries or helped you in your journey to build a stronger *you*, then I would really be grateful if you could leave a review on Amazon.

REFERENCES

A quote by Frank Lloyd Wright. (n.d.). Goodreads. https://www.goodreads.com/quotes/10802-the-longer-i-live-the-more-beautiful-life-becomes-if

A quote by Fred DeVito. (n.d.). Goodreads. https://www.goodreads.com/quotes/646638-if-it-doesn-t-challenge-you-it-doesn-t-change-you

A quote by Jess C. Scott. (n.d.). Goodreads. https://www.goodreads.com/quotes/290462-a-fit-healthy-body-that-is-the-best-fashion-statement

A quote by Mahatma Gandhi. (n.d.). Goodreads. https://www.goodreads.com/quotes/60736-strength-does-not-come-from-physical-capacity-it-comes-from

Alexander, B. H., Rivara, F. P., & Wolf, M. E. (2011). The cost and frequency of hospitalization for fall-related injuries in older adults. *American Journal of Public Health, 82*(7), 1020–1023. https://doi.org/10.2105/ajph.82.7.1020

American Psychological Association. (2020, March 4). *Working out boosts brain health.* Apa.org. https://www.apa.org/topics/exercise-fitness/stress

Aristizabal, J. C., Freidenreich, D. J., Volk, B. M., Kupchak, B. R., Saenz, C., Maresh, C. M., Kraemer, W. J., & Volek, J. S. (2015). Effect of resistance training on resting metabolic rate and its estimation by a dual-energy X-ray absorptiometry metabolic map. *European Journal of Clinical Nutrition, 69,* 831–836. https://doi.org/10.1038/ejcn.2014.216

Arnold Schwarzenegger quotes. (n.d.). BrainyQuote. https://www.brainyquote.com/quotes/arnold_schwarzenegger_166118#

Baig, M. A. & Bordoni, B. (2020). Anatomy, Shoulder and Upper Limb, Pectoral Muscles. PubMed; StatPearls Publishing. https://www.ncbi.nlm.nih.gov/books/NBK545241/

Bailey, R. (n.d.). *How aging affects your joints.* Schiff Vitamins. https://www.schiffvitamins.com/blogs/joint-health/how-aging-affects-your-joints

Barbour, K. E., Helmick, C. G., Boring, M., & Brady, T. J. (2017). Vital signs: Prevalence of doctor-diagnosed arthritis and arthritis-attributable activity limitation—United States, 2013–2015. *Morbidity and Mortality Weekly Report, 66,* 246–253. https://doi.org/10.15585/mmwr.mm6609e1

Bergen, G., Stevens, M. R., & Burns, E. R. (2016). Falls and fall injuries among adults aged ≥65 years—United States, 2014. *MMWR. Morbidity and*

Mortality Weekly Report, 65(37), 993–998. https://doi.org/10.15585/mmwr.mm6537a2

Better Health Channel. (n.d.). *Ageing—muscles bones and joints.* https://www.betterhealth.vic.gov.au/health/conditionsandtreatments/ageing-muscles-bones-and-joints

Blum, C. L. (2019). The many faces of forward head posture: The importance of differential diagnosis. *CRANIO®, 37*(3), 143–146. https://doi.org/10.1080/08869634.2019.1594003

Bontrup, C., Taylor, W. R., Fliesser, M., Visscher, R., Green, T., Wippert, P., & Zemp, R. (2019). Low back pain and its relationship with sitting behaviour among sedentary office workers. *Applied Ergonomics, 81*, 102894. https://doi.org/10.1016/j.apergo.2019.102894

Brown, N., White, J., Brasher, A., & Scurr, J. (2014). An investigation into breast support and sports bra use in female runners of the 2012 London Marathon. *Journal of Sports Sciences, 32*(9), 801–809. https://doi.org/10.1080/02640414.2013.844348

Brumitt, J., & Cuddeford, T. (2015). Current concepts of muscle and tendon adaptation to strength and conditioning. *International Journal of Sports Physical Therapy, 10*(6), 748–759. https://pubmed.ncbi.nlm.nih.gov/26618057/

Cadore, E. L., Rodríguez-Mañas, L., Sinclair, A., & Izquierdo, M. (2013). Effects of different exercise interventions on risk of falls, gait ability, and balance in physically frail older adults: A systematic review. *Rejuvenation Research, 16*(2), 105–114. https://doi.org/10.1089/rej.2012.1397

Cava, E., Yeat, N. C., & Mittendorfer, B. (2017). Preserving healthy muscle during weight loss. *Advances in Nutrition: An International Review Journal, 8*(3), 511–519. https://doi.org/10.3945/an.116.014506

Centers for Disease Control and Prevention. (n.d.). *The truth about aging and dementia.* https://www.cdc.gov/aging/publications/features/dementia-not-normal-aging.html

Celine Dion quotes. (n.d.). BrainyQuote. https://www.brainyquote.com/quotes/celine_dion_457520

Chang, W., Lin, H., & Lai, P. (2015). Core strength training for patients with chronic low back pain. *Journal of Physical Therapy Science, 27*(3), 619–622. https://doi.org/10.1589/jpts.27.619

Chen, J. J., Rosas, H. D., & Salat, D. H. (2011). Age-associated reductions in cerebral blood flow are independent from regional atrophy. *NeuroImage,*

55(2), 468–478. https://doi.org/10.1016/j.neuroimage.2010.12.032

Cleveland Clinic. (n.d.). *Abdominal muscles*. https://my.clevelandclinic.org/health/body/21755-abdominal-muscles

Corpuz, K. (2023, March 7). *This is what skin concerns look like at every age (20s, 30s, 40s, 50s, and beyond)*. Real Simple. https://www.realsimple.com/beauty-fashion/skincare/anti-aging/aging-skin-concerns

Davis, N. (2020, May 29). *If you aren't breathing like this, you're sabotaging your workout*. Healthline. https://www.healthline.com/health/fitness-exercise/when-to-inhale-and-exhale-during-exercise

Demontiero, O., Vidal, C., & Duque, G. (2012). Aging and bone loss: New insights for the clinician. *Therapeutic Advances in Musculoskeletal Disease*, 4(2), 61–76. https://doi.org/10.1177/1759720x11430858

De Ridder, E. M., Van Oosterwijck, J. O., Vleeming, A., Vanderstraeten, G. G., & Danneels, L. A. (2013). Posterior muscle chain activity during various extension exercises: An observational study. *BMC Musculoskeletal Disorders*, 14(1). https://doi.org/10.1186/1471-2474-14-204

Doheny, K. (2021, October 20). *Broken heart syndrome: On the rise, especially in women 50-74*. WebMD. https://www.webmd.com/heart-disease/news/20211020/broken-heart-syndrome-on-rise-middle-age-older-women

Elliot, A. J. (2015). Color and psychological functioning: A review of theoretical and empirical work. *Frontiers in Psychology*, 6(368). https://doi.org/10.3389/fpsyg.2015.00368

Ema, R., Ohki, S., Takayama, H., Kobayashi, Y., & Akagi, R. (2017). Effect of calf-raise training on rapid force production and balance ability in elderly men. *Journal of Applied Physiology*, 123(2), 424–433. https://doi.org/10.1152/japplphysiol.00539.2016

Evans, W. J. (1995). What is sarcopenia? *The Journals of Gerontology Series A: Biological Sciences and Medical Sciences*, 50A, 5–8. https://doi.org/10.1093/gerona/50a.special_issue.5

Evans, W. J. (1999). Exercise training guidelines for the elderly. *Medicine & Science in Sports & Exercise*, 31(1), 12–17. https://doi.org/10.1097/00005768-199901000-00004

Fielding, R. A., Guralnik, J. M., King, A. C., Pahor, M., McDermott, M. M., Tudor-Locke, C., Manini, T. M., Glynn, N. W., Marsh, A. P., Axtell, R. S., Hsu, F.-C., & Rejeski, W. J. (2017). Dose of physical activity, physical functioning and disability risk in mobility-limited older adults: Results from the LIFE study randomized trial. *PLOS ONE*, 12(8). https://doi.org/10.

1371/journal.pone.0182155

Fletcher, J. (2021, January 28). *When and how to spend a rest day.* Medical News Today. https://www.medicalnewstoday.com/articles/rest-day

Fragala, M., Cadore, E., Dorgo, S., Izquierdo, M., Kraemer, W., Peterson, M., & Ryan, E. (2019). *Resistance training for older adults: Position statement from the national strength and conditioning association.* The Journal of Strength and Conditioning Research. https://www.nsca.com/contentassets/2a4112fb355a4a48853bbafbe070fb8e/resistance_training_for_older_adults__position.1.pdf

Frank, P., Andersson, E., Pontén, M., Ekblom, B., Ekblom, M., & Sahlin, K. (2015). Strength training improves muscle aerobic capacity and glucose tolerance in elderly. Scandinavian *Journal of Medicine & Science in Sports, 26*(7), 764–773. https://doi.org/10.1111/sms.12537

Freedman, V. A., & Martin, L. G. (1998). Understanding trends in functional limitations among older Americans. *American Journal of Public Health, 88*(10), 1457–1462. https://doi.org/10.2105/ajph.88.10.1457

Gallegos-Orozco, J. F., Foxx-Orenstein, A. E., Sterler, S. M., & Stoa, J. M. (2012). Chronic constipation in the elderly. *American Journal of Gastroenterology, 107*(1), 18–25. https://doi.org/10.1038/ajg.2011.349

Gordon, B. R., McDowell, C. P., Hallgren, M., Meyer, J. D., Lyons, M., & Herring, M. P. (2018). Association of efficacy of resistance exercise training with depressive symptoms. *JAMA Psychiatry, 75*(6), 566-576. https://doi.org/10.1001/jamapsychiatry.2018.0572

Gordon, B. R., McDowell, C. P., Lyons, M., & Herring, M. P. (2020). Resistance exercise training for anxiety and worry symptoms among young adults: A randomized controlled trial. *Scientific Reports, 10*(1). https://doi.org/10.1038/s41598-020-74608-6

Harvard Health Publishing. (2021, October 13). *Strength training builds more than muscles.* https://www.health.harvard.edu/staying-healthy/strength-training-builds-more-than-muscles

Harvey, J., Chastin, S., & Skelton, D. (2013). Prevalence of sedentary behavior in older adults: A systematic review. *International Journal of Environmental Research and Public Health, 10*(12), 6645–6661. https://doi.org/10.3390/ijerph10126645

Holloszy, J. O. (2000). The biology of aging. *Mayo Clinic Proceedings, 75 Suppl*, S3-8; discussion S8-9. https://pubmed.ncbi.nlm.nih.gov/10959208/

Holloway, B. (2021, November). *The Muscles of the Back.* Goodpath. https://www.goodpath.com/learn/muscles-back

Hotta, K., Kamiya, K., Shimizu, R., Yokoyama, M., Nakamura-Ogura, M., Tabata, M., Kamekawa, D., Akiyama, A., Kato, M., Noda, C., Matsunaga, A., & Masuda, T. (2013). Stretching exercises enhance vascular endothelial function and improve peripheral circulation in patients with acute myocardial infarction. *International Heart Journal, 54*(2), 59–63. https://doi.org/10.1536/ihj.54.59

How aging affects your heart. (n.d.). WebMD. https://www.webmd.com/healthy-aging/ss/slideshow-how-aging-affects-your-heart

Henwood, T. R., Riek, S., & Taaffe, D. R. (2008). Strength versus muscle power-specific resistance training in community-dwelling older adults. *The Journals of Gerontology, 63*(1), 83–91. https://doi.org/10.1093/gerona/63.1.83

Hody, S., Croisier, J., Bury, T., Rogister, B., & Leprince, P. (2019). Eccentric muscle contractions: Risks and benefits. *Frontiers in Physiology, 10,* 536. https://doi.org/10.3389/fphys.2019.00536

Kettinen, J., Tikkanen, H., & Venojärvi, M. (2023). Comparative effectiveness of playing golf to Nordic walking and walking on acute physiological effects on cardiometabolic markers in healthy older adults: A randomised cross-over study. *BMJ Open Sport & Exercise Medicine, 9*(1). https://doi.org/10.1136/bmjsem-2022-001474

Khalil, R. A. (2013). Estrogen, vascular estrogen receptor and hormone therapy in postmenopausal vascular disease. *Biochemical Pharmacology, 86*(12), 1627–1642. https://doi.org/10.1016/j.bcp.2013.09.024

Kirkman, M. S., Briscoe, V. J., Clark, N., Florez, H., Haas, L. B., Halter, J. B., Huang, E. S., Korytkowski, M. T., Munshi, M. N., Odegard, P. S., Pratley, R. E., & Swift, C. S. (2012). Diabetes in older adults. *Diabetes Care, 35*(12), 2650–2664. https://doi.org/10.2337/dc12-1801

Knight, J., & Nigam, Y. (2017). Anatomy and physiology of ageing 5: The nervous system. *Nursing Times, 113*(6), 55–58. https://insights.ovid.com/nursing-times/nrtm/2017/06/000/anatomy-physiology-ageing-nervous-system/13/00006203

Kohn, J. C., Lampi, M. C., & Reinhart-King, C. A. (2015). Age-related vascular stiffening: Causes and consequences. *Frontiers in Genetics, 6.* https://doi.org/10.3389/fgene.2015.00112

Landers, K. A., Hunter, G. R., Wetzstein, C. J., Bamman, M. M., & Weinsier, R.

L. (2001). The interrelationship among muscle mass, strength, and the ability to perform physical tasks of daily living in younger and older women. *The Journals of Gerontology Series A: Biological Sciences and Medical Sciences, 56*(10), B443–B448. https://doi.org/10.1093/gerona/56.10.b443

Landin, D., Thompson, M., & Jackson, M. (2018). Functions of the triceps brachii in humans: A review. *Journal of Clinical Medicine Research, 10*(4), 290–293. https://doi.org/10.14740/jocmr3340w

Landsverk, G. (2021, October 11). *Stop weightlifting in running shoes—they slow your progress and increase your risk of injury.* Insider. https://www.insider.com/stop-weightlifting-in-running-shoes-they-slow-your-progress-expert-2021-10

Latham, N., & Liu, C. (2010). Strength training in older adults: The benefits for osteoarthritis. *Clinics in Geriatric Medicine, 26*(3), 445–459. https://doi.org/10.1016/j.cger.2010.03.006

Lexell, J., Taylor, C. C., & Sjöström, M. (1988). What is the cause of the ageing atrophy? Total number, size and proportion of different fiber types studied in whole vastus lateralis muscle from 15- to 83-year-old men. *Journal of the Neurological Sciences, 84*(2-3), 275–294. https://doi.org/10.1016/0022-510x(88)90132-3

Lord, S., & Castell, S. (1994). Effect of exercise on balance, strength and reaction time in older people. *Australian Journal of Physiotherapy, 40*(2), 83–88. https://doi.org/10.1016/s0004-9514(14)60454-2

Lung, K., St Lucia, K., & Lui, F. (2022). *Anatomy, Thorax, Serratus Anterior Muscles.* PubMed; StatPearls Publishing. https://www.ncbi.nlm.nih.gov/books/NBK531457/

Lye, M. & Donnellan, C. (2000). General cardiology: Heart disease in the elderly. *Heart, 84,* 560–566. https://doi.org/10.1136/heart.84.5.560

Maeo, S., Wu, Y., Huang, M., Sakurai, H., Kusagawa, Y., Sugiyama, T., Kanehisa, H., & Isaka, T. (2022). Triceps brachii hypertrophy is substantially greater after elbow extension training performed in the overhead versus neutral arm position. *European Journal of Sport Science,* 1–26. https://doi.org/10.1080/17461391.2022.2100279

Maiese, K. (2020, April). *Brain, spinal cord, and nerve disorders.* MSD Manual Consumer Version. https://www.msdmanuals.com/en-au/home/brain

Manly, J. J., Jones, R. N., Langa, K. M., Ryan, L. H., Levine, D. A., McCammon, R., Heeringa, S. G., & Weir, D. (2022). Estimating the prevalence of dementia and mild cognitive impairment in the US. JAMA *Neurology,*

79(12) 1242–1249. https://doi.org/10.1001/jamaneurol.2022.3543

Manor, B. (2019, October 22). *Preventing falls in older adults: Multiple strategies are better.* Harvard Health Publishing. https://www.health.harvard.edu/blog/preventing-falls-in-older-adults-multiple-strategies-are-better-2019102218085

Mansi, S., Milosavljevic, S., Baxter, G. D., Tumilty, S., & Hendrick, P. (2014). A systematic review of studies using pedometers as an intervention for musculoskeletal diseases. *BMC Musculoskeletal Disorders, 15*(1). https://doi.org/10.1186/1471-2474-15-231

March, B. (2018, February 1). *7 reasons why what you wear in the gym really matters.* Harper's Bazaar. https://www.harpersbazaar.com/uk/beauty/fitness-wellbeing/a15954030/performance-gym-wear-tips/

Mason, B. R., Page, K.-A., & Fallon, K. (1999). An analysis of movement and discomfort of the female breast during exercise and the effects of breast support in three cases. *Journal of Science and Medicine in Sport, 2*(2), 134–144. https://doi.org/10.1016/S1440-2440(99)80193-5

Mayo Clinic Staff. (2021, October 6). *Aerobic exercise: How to warm up and cool down.* Mayo Clinic. https://www.mayoclinic.org/healthy-lifestyle/fitness/in-depth/exercise/art-20045517?pg=1

McMahon, G. E., Morse, C. I., Burden, A., Winwood, K., & Onambélé, G. L. (2014). Impact of range of motion during ecologically valid resistance training protocols on muscle size, subcutaneous fat, and strength. *Journal of Strength and Conditioning Research, 28*(1), 245–255. https://doi.org/10.1519/jsc.0b013e318297143a

MedlinePlus. (n.d.). *Aging changes in the heart and blood vessels.* https://medlineplus.gov/ency/article/004006.htm

Montagne, A., Barnes, Samuel R., Sweeney, Melanie D., Halliday, Matthew R., Sagare, Abhay P., Zhao, Z., Toga, Arthur W., Jacobs, Russell E., Liu, Collin Y., Amezcua, L., Harrington, Michael G., Chui, Helena C., Law, M., & Zlokovic, Berislav V. (2015). Blood-Brain barrier breakdown in the aging human hippocampus. *Neuron, 85*(2), 296–302. https://doi.org/10.1016/j.neuron.2014.12.032

National Institute on Aging. (n.d.). *Concerned about constipation?* https://www.nia.nih.gov/health/concerned-about-constipation

National Institute on Aging. (n.d.). *Heart health and aging.* https://www.nia.nih.gov/health/heart-health-and-aging

Nieman, D. C., & Wentz, L. M. (2019). The compelling link between physical activity and the body's defense system. *Journal of Sport and Health Science, 8*(3), 201–217. https://doi.org/10.1016/j.jshs.2018.09.009

Nigg, B., Baltich, J., Hoerzer, S., & Enders, H. (2015). Running shoes and running injuries: Mythbusting and a proposal for two new paradigms: "preferred movement path" and "comfort filter." *British Journal of Sports Medicine, 49*(20), 1290–1294. https://doi.org/10.1136/bjsports-2015-095054

Norris, M., Blackmore, T., Horler, B., & Wakefield-Scurr, J. (2021). How the characteristics of sports bras affect their performance. *Ergonomics, 64*(3), 410–425. https://doi.org/10.1080/00140139.2020.1829090

Noto, R. E., Leavitt, L., & Edens, M. A. (2022). Physiology, muscle. National Library of Medicine. https://www.ncbi.nlm.nih.gov/books/NBK532258/

Ohlsson, C., Gidestrand, E., Bellman, J., Larsson, C., Palsdottir, V., Hägg, D., Jansson, P.-A., & Jansson, J.-O. (2020). Increased weight loading reduces body weight and body fat in obese subjects–A proof of concept randomized clinical trial. *EClinicalMedicine, 22*, 100338. https://doi.org/10.1016/j.eclinm.2020.100338

Olivetti, G., Melissari, M., Capasso, J. M., & Anversa, P. (1991). Cardiomyopathy of the aging human heart. Myocyte loss and reactive cellular hypertrophy. *Circulation Research, 68*(6), 1560–1568. https://doi.org/10.1161/01.res.68.6.1560

Opplert, J. & Babault, N. (2017). Acute effects of dynamic stretching on muscle flexibility and performance: An analysis of the current literature. *Sports Medicine, 48*, 299–325. https://doi.org/10.1007/s40279-017-0797-9

Pacifico, J., Geerlings, M. A. J., Reijnierse, E. M., Phassouliotis, C., Lim, W. K., & Maier, A. B. (2020). Prevalence of sarcopenia as a comorbid disease: A systematic review and meta-analysis. *Experimental gerontology, 131*, 110801. https://doi.org/10.1016/j.exger.2019.110801

Paddock, C. (2019, February 21). *Why sleep is good for your arteries.* Medical News Today. https://www.medicalnewstoday.com/articles/324510

Parkkari, J., Kannus, P., Palvanen, M., Natri, A., Vainio, J., Aho, H., Vuori, I., & Järvinen, M. (1999). Majority of hip fractures occur as a result of a fall and impact on the greater trochanter of the femur: A prospective controlled hip fracture study with 206 consecutive patients. *Calcified Tissue International, 65*, 183–187. https://doi.org/10.1007/s002239900679

Raman, R. (2017, September 24). *Why your metabolism slows down with age.* Healthline. https://www.healthline.com/nutrition/metabolism-and-age

Reynolds, G. (2016, July 20). *Lifting lighter weights can be just as effective as heavy ones.* New York Times. https://archive.nytimes.com/well.blogs.nytimes.com/2016/07/20/lifting-lighter-weights-can-be-just-as-effective-as-heavy-ones/

Roubenoff, R. & Castaneda C. (2001). Sarcopenia—Understanding the dynamics of aging muscle. *JAMA, 286*(10), 1230-1231. https://doi.org/10.1001/jama.286.10.1230

Schmall, T. (2021, September 6). *The secret to getting fit is getting new clothes, study finds.* SWNS Media Group. https://www.swnsdigital.com/2018/04/the-secret-to-getting-fit-is-getting-new-clothes-study-finds/

Schoenfeld, B. J., Ogborn, D., & Krieger, J. W. (2016). Effects of resistance training frequency on measures of muscle hypertrophy: A systematic review and meta-analysis. *Sports Medicine, 46*, 1689–1697. https://doi.org/10.1007/s40279-016-0543-8

Schott, N., Johnen, B., & Holfelder, B. (2019). Effects of free weights and machine training on muscular strength in high-functioning older adults. *Experimental Gerontology, 122*, 15–24. https://doi.org/10.1016/j.exger.2019.03.012

Seguin, R., & Nelson, M. E. (2003). The benefits of strength training for older adults. *American Journal of Preventive Medicine, 25*(3), 141–149. https://doi.org/10.1016/s0749-3797(03)00177-6

Seladi-Schulman, J. (2020, April 23). *The causes and symptoms of dehydration in older adults.* Healthline. https://www.healthline.com/health/symptoms-of-dehydration-in-elderly

Shepherd, E., & Brown, T. R. (2016). *Determined, dedicated, disciplined to be fit.* Royal Brown Publishing.

Sions, J. M., Elliott, J. M., Pohlig, R. T., & Hicks, G. E. (2017). Trunk muscle characteristics of the multifidi, erector spinae, psoas, and quadratus lumborum in older adults with and without chronic low back pain. *Journal of Orthopaedic & Sports Physical Therapy, 47*(3), 173–179. https://doi.org/10.2519/jospt.2017.7002

Solari, F. & Burns, B. (2020). *Anatomy, Thorax, Pectoralis Major Major.* PubMed; StatPearls Publishing. https://www.ncbi.nlm.nih.gov/books/NBK525991/

Sole-Smith, V. (2015, October 22). *10 strength-training myths you need to stop believing.* Prevention. https://www.prevention.com/fitness/a20484013/10-strength-training-myths/

Stevens, J. A., Ballesteros, M. F., Mack, K. A., Rudd, R. A., DeCaro, E., & Adler,

G. (2012). Gender differences in seeking care for falls in the aged medicare population. *American Journal of Preventive Medicine, 43*(1), 59–62. https://doi.org/10.1016/j.amepre.2012.03.008

Sundell, J. (2011). Resistance training is an effective tool against metabolic and frailty syndromes. *Advances in Preventive Medicine, 2011*, 1–7. https://doi.org/10.4061/2011/984683

Svennerholm, L., Boström, K., & Jungbjer, B. (1997). Changes in weight and compositions of major membrane components of human brain during the span of adult human life of Swedes. *Acta Neuropathologica, 94*, 345–352. https://doi.org/10.1007/s004010050717

Syed-Abdul, M. M., Soni, D. S., Miller, W. M., Johnson, R. J., Barnes, J. T., Pujol, T. J., & Wagganer, J. D. (2018). Traditional versus suspended push-up muscle activation in athletes and sedentary women. *Journal of Strength and Conditioning Research, 32*(7), 1816–1820. https://doi.org/10.1519/jsc.0000000000002433

Travers, J., Romero-Ortuno, R., Bailey, J., & Cooney, M. (2019). Delaying and reversing frailty: A systematic review of primary care interventions. *British Journal of General Practice, 69*(678), e61–e69. https://doi.org/10.3399/bjgp18x700241

Vellas, B. J., Wayne, S. J., Romero, L. J., Baumgartner, R. N., & Garry, P. J. (1997). Fear of falling and restriction of mobility in elderly fallers. *Age and Ageing, 26*(3), 189–193. https://doi.org/10.1093/ageing/26.3.189

WebMD Editorial Contributors. (n.d.-a). *What to know about dehydration in older adults.* WebMD. https://www.webmd.com/healthy-aging/what-to-know-about-dehydration-in-older-adults

WebMD Editorial Contributors. (n.d-b). *What to know about mental health in older adults.* WebMD. https://www.webmd.com/healthy-aging/mental-health-in-older-adults

Wei, J. Y., & Gersh, B. J. (1987). Heart disease in the elderly. *Current Problems in Cardiology, 12*(1), 1–65. https://pubmed.ncbi.nlm.nih.gov/3549164/

Wewege, M. A., Desai, I., Honey, C., Coorie, B., Jones, M. D., Clifford, B. K., Leake, H. B., & Hagstrom, A. D. (2021). The effect of resistance training in healthy adults on body fat percentage, fat mass and visceral fat: A systematic review and meta-analysis. *Sports Medicine 52*, 287-300. https://doi.org/10.1007/s40279-021-01562-2

Wing, R. R., & Jeffery, R. W. (1999). Benefits of recruiting participants with friends and increasing social support for weight loss and maintenance.

Journal of Consulting and Clinical Psychology, 67(1), 132–138. https://doi.org/10.1037//0022-006x.67.1.132

World Health Organization. (2017, December 12). *Mental health of older adults.* https://www.who.int/news-room/fact-sheets/detail/mental-health-of-older-adults

World Health Organization. (2022, September 20). *Dementia*O. https://www.who.int/news-room/fact-sheets/detail/dementia

Yeun, Y. R. (2017). Effectiveness of resistance exercise using elastic bands on flexibility and balance among the elderly people living in the community: A systematic review and meta-analysis. *Journal of Physical Therapy Science, 29*(9), 1695–1699. https://doi.org/10.1589/jpts.29.1695

Young, W. F. (2022). *Effects of aging on the endocrine system.* MSD Manual Consumer Version. https://www.msdmanuals.com/en-in/home/hormonal-and-metabolic-disorders/biology-of-the-endocrine-system/effects-of-aging-on-the-endocrine-system

Zouita, S., Zouhal, H., Ferchichi, H., Paillard, T., Dziri, C., Hackney, A. C., Laher, I., Granacher, U., & Ben Moussa Zouita, A. (2020). Effects of combined balance and strength training on measures of balance and muscle strength in older women with a history of falls. *Frontiers in Physiology, 11.* https://doi.org/10.3389/fphys.2020.619016

Made in the USA
Middletown, DE
12 April 2025

74149904R00096